GURULIFE

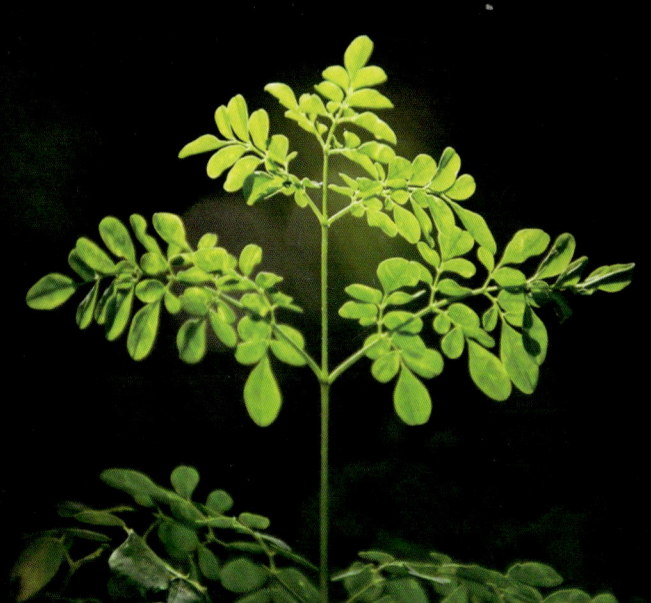

Edition 1
Fall 2017

GURU LIFE
Be Your Own Guru with Natural Protocols to Turn Ailments Into Wellness

1st Edition October 2017

©2017 Guru Wellness Publishing
All rights reserved.

ISBN: 978-0-9993689-1-6

No part of this book may be reproduced or transmitted in any form, or by any means, electronic or mechanical, including photocopy without written permission from the copyright owner.

Published by:

Guru Wellness Publishing
Pleasant Grove, Utah
contact@guruwellnesspublishing.com

Disclaimer to Readers:

This book is intended for reference purposes only. The information contained has not been evaluated by the US Food and Drug Administration, or by other government entities. It is not provided to diagnose, treat, cure, or prevent any disease, illness, or any injured condition of the body.

The authors and publisher of this book are not liable for any misconception or misuse of the information provided. They are not responsible or liable for any person or entity in regards to any damage, loss, or injury caused, or supposed to be caused, either directly or indirectly from the use of the contents of this book.

This book is not intended to be a substitute for medical counseling. Anyone suffering from any illness, injury, or disease should consult a qualified healthcare professional.

About this Book

Be your own GURU. Being the guru of your family's wellness starts with incredible nutrition. This book provides complete, natural protocols for wellness that center around the best nutrition nature has to offer. The information in the protocols and the recommended products come to one point:

You can be your own guru.

No matter your ailment or wellness goal, start with plant-based nutrition. Fuel the body with raw, usable nutrients from Moringa and Moringa-inspired supplements. Then add the powerful effects of versatile essential oils and supplements to enhance and inspire an active lifestyle.

Navigating this book is simple. Look up an ailment in the *Ailments & Conditions* section. Try one or a few of the suggestions for each ailment. Explore the products in the sections that follow.

For the biggest results, you'll find detailed *Protocols* at the end for the 66 most common health ailments. And of course there are a few protocols you can tear out and share with people who want to be their own health gurus too.

Explore the recommendations in this book to discover what works best for you. Creating wellness is a discovery process. What works for one person may not be optimal for another. Play with the protocols, and have fun becoming your own guru.

Table of Contents

Section 1
Wellness Revolution & Usage Guide......................pg.7

Section 2
Ailments & Conditions......................................pg.11

Section 3
Nutritionals..pg.47

Section 4
Single Oils..pg.67

Section 5
Oil Blends..pg.113

Section 6
Protocols..pg.141

Bibliography..pg.165

Section 7
Tear-out Protocols to Share..............................pg.167

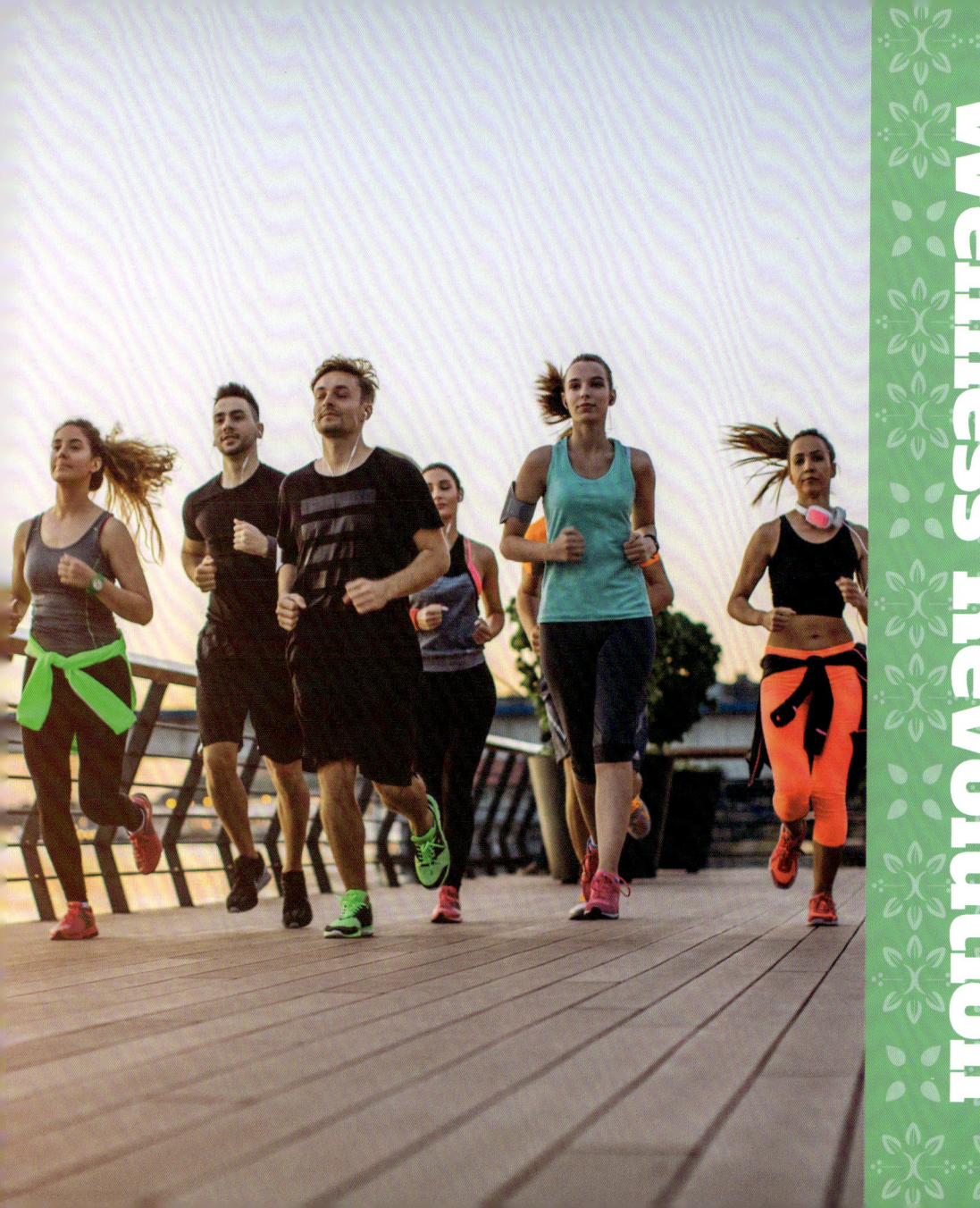

Wellness Revolution

Ingredients
for a total wellness revolution

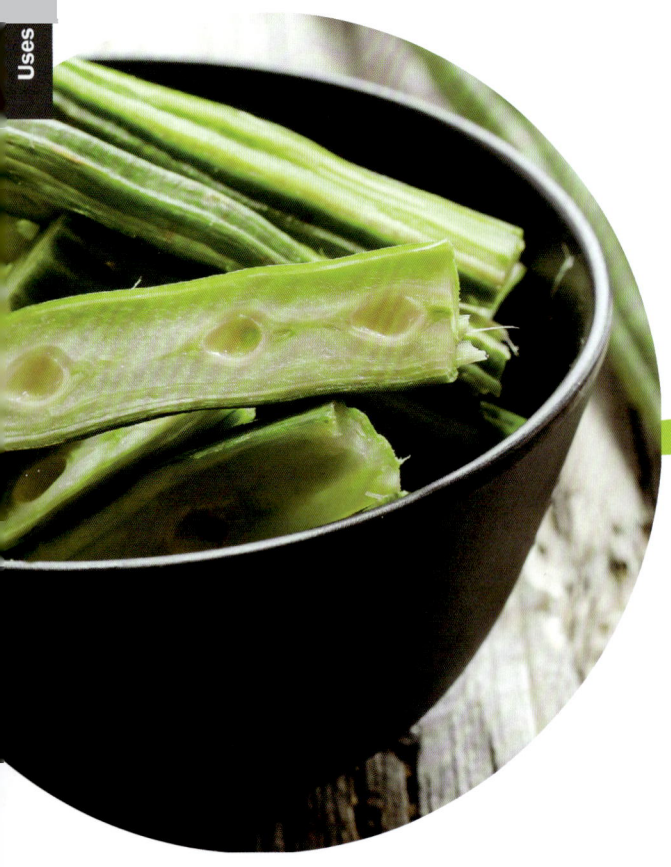

✺ Moringa Oleifera Powder
Start with a core of Moringa nutrition.

Your body wants incredible nutrition. Moringa is the perfect center to properly fueling the cells of your body.

A serving of moringa powder contains over 90 verifiable, cell-ready vitamins, minerals, crucial proteins, antioxidants, omega fatty acids, and plenty of other benefits.

Once you've got the center for your revolution, then you can add on the right things to tailor it to your specific needs.

Uses

Essential Oils

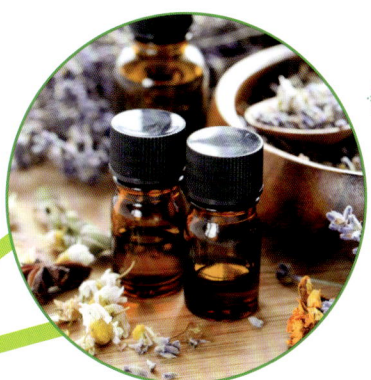

Use essential oils to target specific health needs. They're versatile, and work on the level of both symptoms and root causes.

Skincare

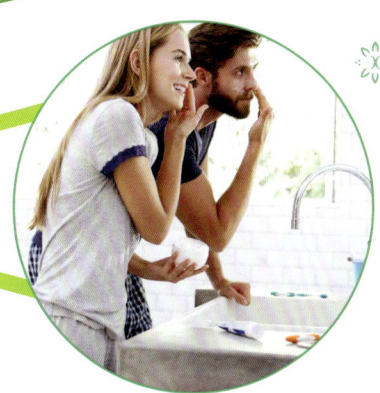

Avoid toxic chemicals by using plant-based skincare & beauty products. Feel healthy on the inside and outside.

Fitness Fuel

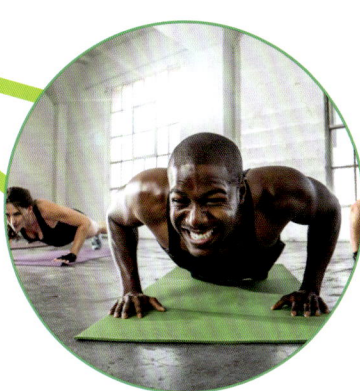

Support your health by fueling an active lifestyle. Smart supplements mean more energy and faster recovery, and more motivation to take care of your body.

Usage & Safety

Moringa powder and workout powders have one way to use them: Drink them. Essential oils, on the other hand, are versatile and can be used many ways. If you know your oils have undergone stringent testing and are verified to be pure, use them in these ways:

Aromatic
Inhale a few drops from your palms, or use several drops in a diffuser. Aromatic use is ideal for respiratory, mental, and emotional needs.

Topical
Apply directly to skin (neat), or apply diluted with a carrier oil. It's always safe to apply oils to the bottoms of feet if you can't apply an oil directly the affected area.

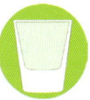

Internal
If an oil has supplement facts on the bottle, drink a couple drops in water or in a veggie capsule. Internal use provides quick effects and full-body delivery.

Cautions
While pure oils are extremely safe for everyone, use caution when pregnant, epileptic, or dealing with other major health concerns. Each oil in this book will have a safety note if it should be used with caution or avoided under certain conditions.

Dilute oils with a carrier oil for children and people with sensitive skin.
- Babies 1:30 (1 part oil, 30 parts carrier oil)
- Toddlers 1:20
- Children 1:10
- Adults 1:(dilute according to preference)

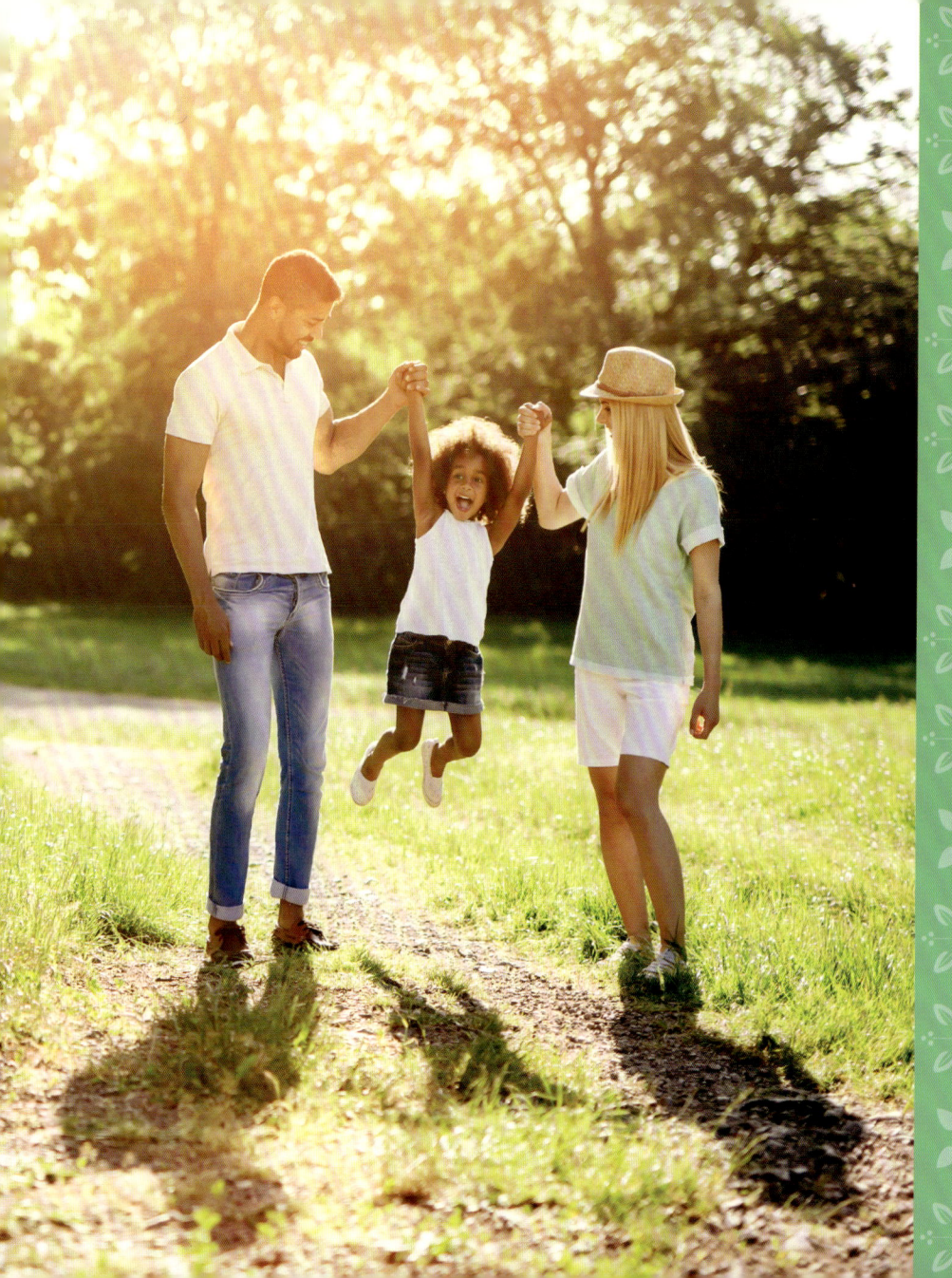

Ailments & Conditions

Ailments

Acid Reflux
Digestive Support Blend [TI]
Peppermint [TI]
Ginger [TI]
Nutmeg [TI]
Coriander [TI]

Take 2-4 drops of oil internally or apply to stomach area as needed.

Protocol on pg. 154

Acne/Blemishes
Use Premium Tea to cleanse the body. Apply a drop topically to affected areas. Add 2-3 drops to lotion and apply after cleansing routine.

Premium Tea [I]
Skin-Enriching Blend [T]
Tea Tree [TI]
Lavender [TI]
Eucalyptus [TI]

Protocol on pg. 142

ADD/ADHD
Moringa Super Powder [I]
Focusing Blend [AT]
Concentration Blend [AT]
Vetiver [ATI]
Frankincense [ATI]

Use Moringa daily. Apply a few drops of oil on forehead and back of neck; inhale a few drops from cupped hands.

Adrenal Fatigue
Use the energy mix morning and afternoon. Massage 1-3 drops of oil on lower back over adrenals, or inhale from cupped hands; ingest 1-3 drops as needed.

Extreme Moringa Energy [I]
Limitless Energy Powder [I]
Basil [ATI]
Rosemary [ATI]
Peppermint [ATI]

Protocol on pg. 143

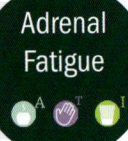

Aging
Optimal Aging Formula [I]
Frankincense [TI]
Atlas Cedarwood [TI]
Sandalwood [TI]
Antioxidant Blend [TI]

Use aging formula as directed. Apply 1-3 drops of oil to target areas. Combine 2-8 drops with facial lotion or carrier oil and apply after cleansing.

Alertness
Use Moringa energy and/or nitric oxide activator. Apply oils to forehead, on temples, or base of skull as needed; inhale a few drops from cupped hands.

Extreme Moringa Energy [I]
Nitric Oxide Activator [I]
Basil [ATI]
Rosemary [ATI]
Peppermint [ATI]

Allergies (seasonal)
Lavender [ATI]
Peppermint [ATI]
Respiration Blend [AT]
Respiratory Blend [AT]
Detoxification Blend [ATI]

Apply to back of neck, under nose, on bridge of nose, or over chest as needed. Take a few drops internally or diffuse several drops.

Protocol on pg. 144

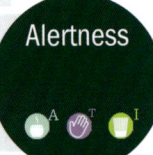

Alzheimer's & Dementia
Use nitric oxide activator and Moringa. Massage 1-2 drops of oil into scalp once daily. Ingest 2-4 drops 1-2 times daily.

Nitric Oxide Activator [I]
Moringa Super Powder [I]
Frankincense [ATI]
Rosemary [ATI]
Antioxidant Blend [ATI]

Protocol on pg. 144

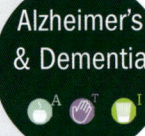

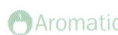 Aromatic   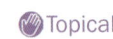 Topical   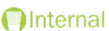 Internal

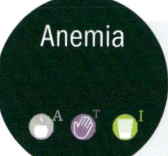

Anemia

Moringa Super Powder [I]
Protecting Blend [T I]
Basil [T I]
Lemon [T I]
Lavender [T I]

Use Moringa daily. Apply 1-3 drops of oil to bottoms of feet and inside of wrists; take a few drops internally; or inhale from cupped hands periodically.

Use caps in the morning or before exercise. Apply 1-3 drops of oil to temples and/or chest; inhale a few drops from cupped hands as needed.

AM Exercise Caps [I]
Stress Control Blend [A T]
Comforting Blend [A T]
Concentration Blend [A T]
Lemongrass [A T I]

Anger

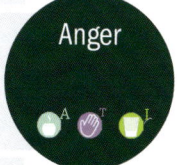

Ankle Swelling

Juniper Berry [T I]
Cypress [T]
Lemongrass [T I]
Soothing Blend [T]
Balsam Fir [T I]

Massage ankles with 2-4 drops, diluted with carrier oil if desired.

Use Moringa and tea. Apply 1-3 drops of oil to stomach area, or inhale from cupped hands as needed.

Moringa Super Powder [I]
Premium Tea [I]
Weight Control Blend [A T I]
Slimming Blend [A T I]
Vitality-Boosting Blend [A T I]

Anorexia

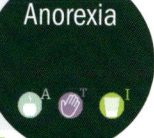

Anxiety

Nitric Oxide Activator [I]
Vetiver [A T I]
Balancing Blend [A T]
Lavender [A T I]
Stress Control Blend [A T]

Use nitric oxide activator. Apply 1-3 drops of oil to bottoms of feet, chest, or temples, or inhale from cupped hands as needed.

Protocol on pg. 145

Use nitric oxide activator or energy powder. Apply 1-3 drops of oil to bottoms of feet, chest, or temples, or inhale from cupped hands as needed.

Nitric Oxide Activator [I]
Limitless Energy Powder [I]
Vitality-Boosting Blend [A T I]
Patchouli [A T I]
Myrtle [A T I]

Apathy

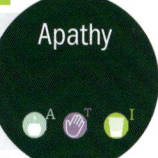

Appetite Suppressant

Extreme Moringa Energy [I]
Premium Tea [I]
PM Craving Control Caps [I]
Slimming Blend [A T I]
Weight Control Blend [A T I]

Use Moringa, tea, and caps daily. Apply 1-3 drops of oil to stomach, chest, bottoms of feet, or inside of wrists, or take 2-4 drops internally.

Protocol on pg. 145

Use aging formula. Massage 1-3 drops of oil into affected areas with lotion or carrier oil as needed.

Optimal Aging Formula [I]
Soothing Blend [A T]
Copaiba [A T I]
Massage Blend [A T]
Wintergreen [A T]

Arthritic Pain

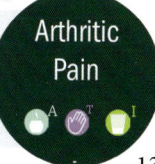

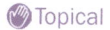 Aromatic   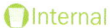 Topical   Internal

13

Ailments

Asthma
Respiratory Blend [A T]
Eucalyptus [A T I]
Rosemary [A T I]
German Chamomile [A T I]
Bergamot [A T I]

Apply 1-3 drops of oil topically to chest, neck, under nose, and on lung reflex points, or inhale from cupped hands as needed.

Protocol on pg. 145

Athlete's Foot
Apply 1-3 drops to area between toes and around toenails 2-3 times daily. Ingest 1-3 drops of Tea Tree or Oregano once a day.

Tea Tree [T I]
Oregano [T I]
Nourishing Blend [T I]
Spruce [T]
Eucalyptus [T I]

Autism/Asperger's
Moringa Super Powder [I]
Frankincense [A T I]
Geranium [A T I]
Purifying Blend [A T]
Concentration Blend [A T]

Use Moringa. Apply 1-3 drops of oil to bottoms of feet and back of neck. Ingest 1-3 drops of Cilantro and Frankincense 1-2 times daily.

Protocol on pg. 146

Autoimmune Disorders
Use Moringa and aging formula. Apply 1-3 drops of oil to stomach, chest, bottoms of feet, or inside of wrists. Ingest 1-3 drops daily for added support.

Moringa Super Powder [I]
Optimal Aging Formula [I]
Antioxidant Blend [A T I]
Frankincense [A T I]
Ginger [A T I]

Auto-intoxication
Premium Tea [I]
Detoxification Blend [T I]
Antioxidant Blend [T I]
Digestive Support Blend [T I]
Oregano [T I]

Use Premium Tea. Apply 1-3 drops of oil to stomach, chest, bottoms of feet, or inside of wrists. Ingest 1-3 drops 2-3 times daily for additional support.

Back Pain
Use nitric oxide activator and thermogenic caps to increase blood flow. Massage 2-4 drops of oil into affected areas as needed.

Protocol on pg. 146

Advanced Thermogenic Caps [I]
Nitric Oxide Activator [I]
Soothing Blend [A T]
Massage Blend [A T]
Copaiba [A T I]

Bacterial Infection
Thyme [T I]
Oregano [T I]
Protecting Blend [T I]
Tea Tree [T I]
Roman Chamomile [T I]

Apply 1-3 drops with a carrier oil to the affected areas as needed. Ingest 1-3 drops every 2-3 hours for systemic and/or internal infections.

Balance Problems
Use nitric oxide activator. Apply 1-3 drops of oil to temples, back of neck, and behind the ears, or inhale from cupped hands. Ingest 1-3 drops of ginger as needed.

Nitric Oxide Activator [I]
Ginger [A T I]
Peppermint [A T I]
Basil [A T I]
Balancing Blend [A T]

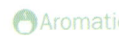 Aromatic 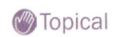 Topical 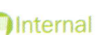 Internal

Bed-Wetting

Cypress [A T]
Black Pepper [A T I]
Ylang Ylang [A T I]
Lemongrass [A T I]
Roman Chamomile [A T I]

Massage 1-3 drops over bladder and kidneys before bedtime as needed.

Apply 1-2 drops topically to sting several times daily until symptoms cease.

Lavender [T I]
Roman Chamomile [T I]
Basil [T I]
Lemongrass [T I]
Skin-Enriching Blend [T]

Bee Sting

Bell's Palsy

Extreme Moringa Caps [I]
Nitric Oxide Activator [I]
Lemongrass [T I]
Frankincense [T I]
Thyme [T I]

Use capsules and activator. Ingest 1-3 drops of oil every 2-3 hours as needed.

Use Moringa. Apply 1-3 drops of oil to bottoms of feet, chest, or temples, or inhale from cupped hands as needed.

Moringa Super Powder [I]
Focusing Blend [A T]
Frankincense [A T I]
Vetiver [A T I]
Tangerine [A T I]

Bipolar Disorder

Bladder Control

Juniper Berry [A T I]
Rosemary [A T I]
Cypress [A T]
Lavender [A T I]
Sandalwood [A T I]

Apply 1-3 drops topically over bladder and kidneys. Add 1-2 drops to drinking water if desired.

Apply a drop topically to affected area as needed.

Helichrysum [T I]
Myrrh [T I]
Geranium [T I]
Lemon [T I]
Tea Tree [T I]

Bleeding

Blisters

Frankincense [T]
Patchouli [T]
Tea Tree [T]
Lavender [T]
Myrrh [T]

Apply a few drops topically to affected area.

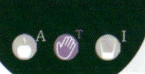 Protocol on pg. 153

Use tea as needed. Apply 1-3 drops of oil to stomach, rubbing in a clockwise direction. Ingest 1-3 drops internally as needed.

Premium Tea [I]
Digestive Support Blend [T I]
Coriander [T I]
Fennel [T I]
Peppermint [T I]

Bloating

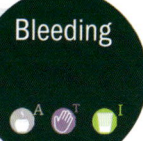

Ailments

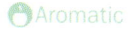 Aromatic 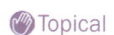 Topical 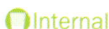 Internal

15

Ailments

Blood Clotting
Advanced Thermogenic Caps [I]
Cypress [T]
Clove [T I]
Marjoram [T I]
Basil [T I]

Use caps once or twice daily. Apply 1-3 drops of oil to bottoms of feet, or ingest a few drops internally as needed.

Blood Pressure (high)
Protocol on pg. 147

Use tea once or twice daily. Apply 2-4 drops of oil to bottoms of feet, or ingest 1-3 drops as needed.

Daily Tea [I]
Marjoram [A T I]
Lemon [A T I]
Cypress [A T]
Ylang Ylang [A T I]

Blood Pressure (low)
Advanced Thermogenic Caps [I]
Helichrysum [T I]
Cypress [T]
Thyme [T I]

Use caps once or twice daily. Apply 2-4 drops of oil to bottoms of feet, or ingest 1-3 drops as needed.

Blood Sugar (low)
Drink workout powder for a pick-me-up. Apply 1-3 drops of oil to stomach or over pancreas, or ingest 1-3 drops as needed.

During Workout Powder [I]
Fennel [T I]
Cinnamon [T I]
Orange [T I]
Coriander [T I]

Blurred Vision
Optimal Aging Formula [I]
Clary Sage [T]
Lemongrass [T]
Helichrysum [T]
Skin-Enriching Blend [T]

Use aging formula daily. Mix desired oils in a roller bottle with carrier oil and carefully apply around eyes 2-4 times daily.

Body Odor
Protocol on pg. 151

Take 1-3 drops of Cilantro, Detoxification Blend, or Geranium at least once daily. Apply 1-3 drops on bottoms of feet.

Premium Tea [I]
Coriander [T I]
Detoxification Blend [T I]
Scotch Pine [T I]
Geranium [T I]

Boils
Skin-Enriching Blend [T]
Tea Tree [T]
Lavender [T]
Myrrh [T]
Bergamot [T]

Apply 1-3 drops topically to affected areas several times daily.

Bone Pain or Break
Use Moringa to supply needed nutrients. Apply 1-3 drops of oil topically to affected areas as needed. Massage with lotion or carrier oil to improve efficacy.

Moringa Super Powder [I]
Soothing Blend [T]
Wintergreen [T]
Helichrysum [T I]

16

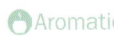 Aromatic   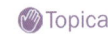 Topical   Internal

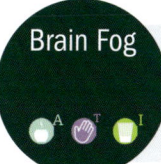

Brain Fog

Nitric Oxide Activator [I]
Frankincense [A T I]
Vitality-Boosting Blend [A T I]
Focusing Blend [A T]
Basil [A T I]

Use activator as needed. Apply 1-3 drops of oil to forehead, temples, back of neck, and behind ears, or inhale from cupped hands as needed.

Use Extreme Moringa Caps. Apply a few drops of oil topically to forehead, temples, base of skull, and behind the ears, or diffuse. Take a few drops internally as needed.

Extreme Moringa Caps [I]
Frankincense [A T I]
Nourishing Blend [A T I]
Balancing Blend [A T]
Sandalwood [A T I]

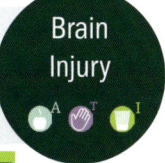

Brain Injury

Breastfeeding (increase milk)

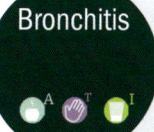

Moringa Super Powder [I]
Fennel [T I]
Basil [T I]
Fennel [T I]
Women's Daily Balancing [I]

Use Moringa Super Powder to supply needed nutrients. Massage 1-3 drops with carrier oil over breasts and apply to bottoms of feet, or take internally when needed.

Protocol on pg. 158

Use Moringa Super Powder for long term benefit. Apply 1-2 drops of oil to nail bed once or twice daily.

Moringa Super Powder [I]
Myrrh [T]
Fennel [T]
Copaiba [T]
Tea Tree [T]

Brittle Nails

Bronchitis

Extreme Moringa Energy [I]
Respiratory Blend [A T]
Black Pepper [A T I]
Respiration Blend [A T]
Lime [A T I]

Use Moringa energy mix to boost immune system. Apply 1-3 drops of oil to chest, gargle hourly, or inhale from cupped hands as needed.

Protocol on pg. 147

Apply 1-3 drops to bruise area. Use carrier oil if desired. Reapply 2-4 times daily.

Restorative Blend [T]
Wintergreen [T]
Cypress [T]
Soothing Blend [T]
Helichrysum [T]

Bruising

Bunions

Copaiba [T]
Lemon [T]
Soothing Blend [T]
Ginger [T]
Cypress [T]

Apply 1-3 drops with carrier oil to affected area or joint as needed.

Use aging formula to provide nutrients to skin. Apply 1-3 drops of oil to affected area hourly or as needed.

Optimal Aging Formula [T]
Lavender [T]
Helichrysum [T]
Skin-Enriching Blend [T]
Atlas Cedarwood [T]

Burns

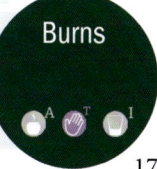

Aromatic   Topical   Internal

Ailments

Cancer
Moringa Super Powder[I]
Nourishing Blend[ATI]
Frankincense[ATI]
Sandalwood[ATI]
Patchouli[ATI]

Use Moringa. Ingest 1-3 drops of oil at least twice daily, and apply topically as close to the affected area as possible.

Protocol on pg. 148

Candida
Apply 1-3 drops to affected area or ingest 1-3 drops at least twice daily until symptoms subside.

Protocol on pg. 148

Immunity-Boosting Blend[TI]
Thyme[TI]
Oregano[TI]
Tea Tree[TI]
Rosemary[TI]

Canker Sores
Extreme Moringa Energy[I]
Tea Tree[TI]
Protecting Blend[TI]
Oregano[TI]
Frankincense[TI]

Use Moringa energy mix to boost immune system. Apply a drop of oil diluted directly to canker sore, or gargle several times daily until sore is gone.

Protocol on pg. 148

Cardiovascular Disease
Use activator daily. Apply 1-3 drops of oil to chest or ingest 1-3 drops as needed.

Nitric Oxide Activator[I]
Antioxidant Blend[TI]
Geranium[TI]
Tangerine[TI]
Cypress[T]

Carpal Tunnel
Moringa Super Powder[I]
Soothing Blend[AT]
Wintergreen[AT]
Lemongrass[ATI]
Marjoram[ATI]

Use Moringa to supply needed nutrients. Apply 1-3 drops of oil to affected area several times daily. Massage with carrier oil or lotion for improved efficacy.

Cartilage Injury
Apply 1-3 drops to affected area several times daily. Massage with carrier oil or lotion for improved efficacy.

Soothing Blend[T]
Lemongrass[TI]
Helichrysum[TI]
Frankincense[TI]
Copaiba[TI]

Cavities
Clove[TI]
Protecting Blend[TI]
Tea Tree[TI]

Apply 1-2 drops directly to tooth. Dilute with carrier oil if necessary.

Cellulite (fat deposits)
Use caps to enhance and encourage exercise. Massage 4-8 drops of oil on target areas daily, especially before exercising. Add to drinking water throughout the day.

Protocol on pg. 163

Advanced Thermogenic Caps[I]
AM Exercise Caps[I]
Slimming Blend[TI]
Weight Control Blend[TI]
Grapefruit[TI]

18

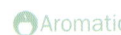 Aromatic   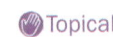 Topical   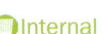 Internal

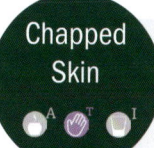
Chapped Skin

Moringa Skincare Products [T]
Myrrh [T]
Skin-Enriching Blend [T]
Atlas Cedarwood [T]
Frankincense [T]

Nourish skin with Moringa-enhanced skincare. Apply a drop or two of oil to affected area as often as needed. Use a carrier oil to increase efficacy.

Use nitric oxide activator. Massage 1-3 drops of oil on area of concern. Use a carrier oil or lotion for improved efficacy.

Nitric Oxide Activator [I]
Massage Blend [T]
Soothing Blend [T]
Marjoram [T,I]
Black Pepper [T,I]

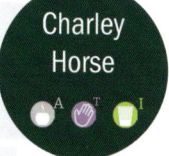
Charley Horse

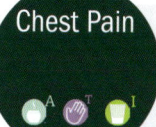
Chest Pain

Premium Tea [I]
Nourishing Blend [A,T,I]
Rosemary [A,T,I]
Orange [A,T,I]
Marjoram [A,T,I]

Use tea to sooth nerves. Apply 1-3 drops of oil topically to chest or ingest at least twice daily.

Use Moringa to boost immune system. Dilute 2-4 drops with a carrier oil and dab lightly on spots a couple times a day; ingest for immune support.

Moringa Super Powder [I]
Thyme [T,I]
Tea Tree [T,I]
Detoxification Blend [T,I]
Eucalyptus [T,I]

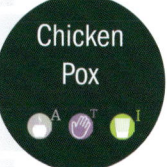
Chicken Pox

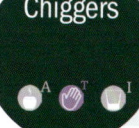
Chiggers

Atlas Cedarwood [T]
Lemongrass [T]
Tea Tree [T]
Detoxification Blend [T]
Purifying Blend [T]

Dilute 2-4 drops with a carrier oil and dab lightly on bites a couple times a day.

Protocol on pg. 149

Use nitric oxide activator. Apply 1-3 drops of oil to chest area or bottoms of feet; ingest 2-4 drops once daily.

Nitric Oxide Activator [I]
Slimming Blend [T,I]
Lavender [T,I]
Cypress [T,I]
Rosemary [T,I]

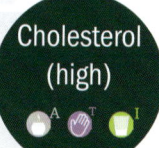
Cholesterol (high)

Chronic Fatigue

Moringa Super Powder [I]
AM Exercise Caps [I]
Vitality-Boosting Blend [A,T,I]
Peppermint [A,T,I]
Basil [A,T,I]

Use Moringa and caps daily. Apply 2-4 drops of oil to bottoms of feet and over adrenals. Also inhale 1-3 drops from cupped hands.

Protocol on pg. 153

Use Moringa and nitric oxide activator. Apply 1-3 drops of oil to affected areas as needed, or use internally under the tongue as needed.

Nitric Oxide Activator [I]
Moringa Super Powder [I]
Soothing Blend [A,T]
Copaiba [A,T,I]
Frankincense [A,T,I]

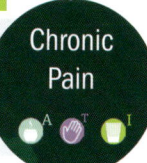
Chronic Pain

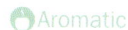 Aromatic 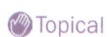 Topical 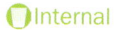 Internal

Ailments

Circulation Issues
Nitric Oxide Activator [I]
Cypress [T]
Ginger [T I]
Black Pepper [T I]
Basil [T I]

Use nitric oxide activator. Apply 1-3 drops of oil to bottoms of feet; ingest 1-3 drops twice daily, or as needed.

Colds
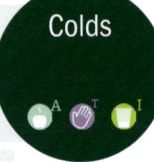

Protocol on pg. 150

Use Moringa energy mix to boost immune system. Ingest 1-3 drops of oil 3-6 times until symptoms subside; rub 2-4 drops on bottoms of feet.

Extreme Moringa Energy [I]
Protecting Blend [A T I]
Immunity-Boosting Blend [A T I]
Oregano [A T I]
Thyme [A T I]

Cold Extremities
Nitric Oxide Activator [I]
Cinnamon [T I]
Black Pepper [T I]
Protecting Blend [T I]
Cypress [T]

Use nitric oxide activator. Apply 1-3 of oil drops to bottoms of feet, chest area, and inside of wrists; ingest 2-4 drops daily as needed.

Cold Sores
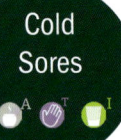

Protocol on pg. 150

Use Moringa daily to keep immune system high. Apply a drop of oil diluted to affected area as needed.

Moringa Super Powder [I]
Protecting Blend [T I]
Tea Tree [T I]
Clove [T I]
Frankincense [T I]

Colic
Roman Chamomile [T]
Marjoram [T]
Bergamot [T]
Coriander [T]
Lemon [T]

Dilute 1-2 drops with a carrier oil and apply topically to stomach and back before baby goes to sleep.

Use nitric oxide activator. Apply 2-4 drops of oil to forehead and base of skull; inhale 1-3 drops from cupped hands; take 1-3 drops internally for a few days.

Nitric Oxide Activator [I]
Frankincense [A T I]
Cypress [A T]
Copaiba [A T I]
Rosemary [A T I]

Concussion
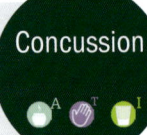

Congestion
Peppermint [A T I]
Respiration Blend [A T]
Eucalyptus [A T I]
Lime [A T I]
Scotch Pine [A T]

Apply 1-3 drops to back of neck, under nose, on bridge of nose, or chest; inhale 1-3 drops from cupped hands as needed.

Protocol on pg. 153

Use tea 1-2 times daily. Massage 1-3 drops of oil over abdomen. Repeat as desired every 5-10 minutes until condition improves.

Premium Tea [I]
Digestive Support Blend [T I]
Ginger [T I]
Lemongrass [T I]
Fennel [T I]

Constipation
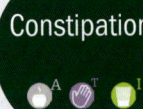

Aromatic   Topical   Internal

20

Cortisol (heightened)

Premium Tea [I]
Lavender [ATI]
Ylang Ylang [ATI]
Rosemary [ATI]
Coriander [ATI]

Use tea as directed. Apply 1-3 drops of oil to back of neck, under nose, on bridge of nose, or chest as needed; ingest 2-4 drops; inhale from cupped hands.

Protocol on pg. 161

Cough

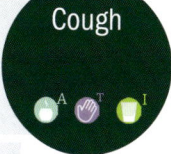

Protocol on pg. 150

Use nitric oxide activator to stimulate immune system. Apply 1-3 drops of oil to chest, back of neck, under nose, or on bridge of nose; inhale from cupped hands.

Nitric Oxide Activator [I]
Respiratory Blend [AT]
Respiration Blend [AT]
Lemon [ATI]
Rosemary [ATI]

Cramps

Post-Workout Powder [I]
Soothing Blend [AT]
Cypress [AT]
Monthly Blend [AT]
Massage Blend [AT]

Use post-workout powder to restore the body. Massage 1-3 drops of oil into affected areas as needed. Use with carrier oil to improve efficacy.

Croup

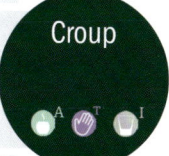

Dilute with carrier oil and apply 1-3 drops to baby's chest and back as needed. Diffuse several drops.

Atlas Cedarwood [AT]
Lemon [AT]
Respiration Blend [AT]
Sandalwood [AT]
Orange [AT]

Crying

Lavender [AT]
Orange [AT]
Comforting Blend [AT]
Roman Chamomile [AT]
Stress-Control Blend [AT]

Apply 1-2 drops to front of shirt or sleeve, or diffuse.

Cuts

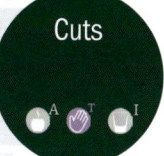

Dilute 1-2 drops with a carrier oil and apply to affected area a couple times daily.

Lavender [T]
Myrrh [T]
Tea Tree [T]
Helichrysum [T]
Atlas Cedarwood [T]

Cystic Fibrosis

Nitric Oxide Activator [I]
Sandalwood [ATI]
Respiration Blend [AT]
Myrrh [ATI]
Roman Chamomile [ATI]

Use nitric oxide activator. Apply 1-3 drops of oil to chest and under nose; inhale from cupped hands as needed.

Apply 1-2 drops to affected area daily or as needed.

Frankincense [TI]
Nourishing Blend [TI]
Oregano [TI]
Tangerine [TI]
Protecting Blend [TI]

Cysts

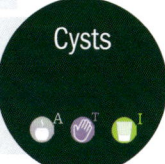

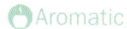 Aromatic 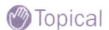 Topical 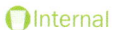 Internal

Ailments

Ailments

Dandruff
Atlas Cedarwood [T]
Tea Tree [T]
Rosemary [T]
Myrrh [T]
Wintergreen [T]

Dilute 2-6 drops in carrier oil and massage into scalp. Rinse after 60 minutes.

Dehydrated Skin
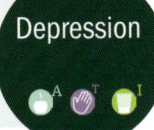

Use Moringa-enhanced skincare. Apply 1-3 drops of oil with carrier oil to affected area as needed. Use with lotion for improved efficacy.

Moringa Skincare Products [T]
Sandalwood [T]
Myrrh [T]
Blue Tansy [T]
Coriander [T]

Dementia
Nitric Oxide Activator [ATI]
Frankincense [ATI]
Nourishing Blend [ATI]
Rosemary [ATI]
Peppermint [ATI]

Use nitric oxide activator. Apply 1-3 drops of oil to base of skull and behind the ears; take internally as needed; inhale from cupped hands as needed.

Protocol on pg. 144

Depression
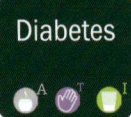

Use Moringa 1-2 times daily. Apply 1-3 drops of oil to forehead and temples; place a drop of frankincense on thumb and press to roof of mouth; inhale from cupped hands.

Moringa Super Powder [I]
Myrtle [ATI]
Spearmint [ATI]
Frankincense [ATI]
Vitality-Boosting Blend [ATI]

Protocol on pg. 151

Detoxification
Premium Tea [I]
Detoxification Blend [TI]
Antioxidant Blend [TI]
Lemongrass [TI]
Clove [TI]

Use tea daily. Apply 3-5 drops of oil to bottoms of feet and inside of wrists; ingest 2-4 drops a few times daily; supplement regularly for improved cleansing.

Protocol on pg. 152

Diabetes
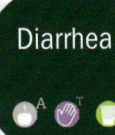

Use tea and caps daily. Apply a couple drops over pancreas and bottoms of feet daily; take a few drops internally.

Premium Tea [I]
PM Craving Control Caps [I]
Cinnamon [TI]
Coriander [TI]
Juniper Berry [TI]

Protocol on pg. 152

Diaper Rash
Lavender [T]
Roman Chamomile [T]
Ylang Ylang [T]
Coriander [T]
Atlas Cedarwood [T]

Dilute 1-3 drops with carrier oil and apply to affected area several times daily until rash disappears.

Diarrhea
Ingest 2-4 drops of oil; massage 1-3 drops into abdomen clockwise hourly as needed. Use hydration powder to replenish body.

Digestive Support Blend [TI]
Coriander [TI]
Ginger [TI]
Patchouli [TI]
Hydration Powder [I]

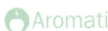 Aromatic 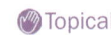 Topical 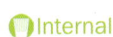 Internal

Diverticulitis
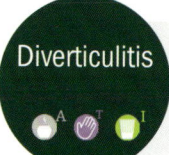

Digestive Support Blend [TI]
Basil [TI]
Nourishing Blend [TI]
Helichrysum [TI]
Frankincense [TI]

Ingest 2-4 drops twice daily to reduce inflammation; massage 1-3 drops into abdomen. Use Frankincense & Helichrysum internally for long-term healing.

Dizziness

Use nitric oxide activator. Apply 1-3 drops of oil to back of neck or on temples; inhale from cupped hands; ingest 2-4 drops of Antioxidant Blend as needed.

Nitric Oxide Activator [I]
Balancing Blend [AT]
Cypress [AT]
Atlas Cedarwood [ATI]
Antioxidant Blend [ATI]

Drug Addiction

PM Craving Control Caps [I]
Detoxification Blend [ATI]
Cinnamon [ATI]
Black Pepper [ATI]
Weight Control Blend [ATI]

Use caps throughout the day. Apply a couple drops of oil to chest, temples, and bottoms of feet daily; inhale from cupped hands as needed.

Dysentery

Use tea to soothe the gut. Massage 1-3 drops of oil into abdomen; ingest 2-4 drops as needed.

Daily Tea [I]
Ginger [TI]
Myrrh [TI]
Eucalyptus Globulus [TI]
Scotch Pine [T]

Dysphagia

Ginger [TI]
Black Pepper [TI]
Fennel [TI]
Peppermint [TI]
Lavender [TI]

Apply 1-3 drops to neck or ingest a few drops as needed.

Ear Infection

Use Moringa to boost immune system. Apply 1-3 drops of oil around the opening of the ear, or apply to a cotton ball. Do NOT use essential oils in ear.

Moringa Super Powder [I]
Basil [TI]
Tea Tree [TI]
Rosemary [TI]
Thyme [TI]

Earache

Helichrysum [TI]
Basil [TI]
Ginger [TI]
Spruce [TI]
Lavender [TI]

Apply 1-3 drops of oil around the opening of the ear, or apply to a cotton ball and rest over ear for 15 minutes. Do NOT use essential oils in ear.

Eczema

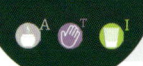
Protocol on pg. 153

Use tea and aging formula to cleanse and replenish the system. Apply 2-4 drops of oil to affected area as needed. Dilute as needed.

Premium Tea [I]
Optimal Aging Formula [I]
Skin-Enriching Blend [TI]
Helichrysum [TI]
Atlas Cedarwood [TI]

Ailments

Aromatic · Topical · Internal

23

Ailments

Edema
Juniper Berry [TI]
Cypress [T]
Lemongrass [TI]
Slimming Blend [TI]
Grapefruit [TI]

Massage 1-3 drops into affected area and on bottoms of feet; ingest a couple times daily or as needed.

Emphysema
Apply 1-3 drops to back of neck, under nose, chest, or on bridge of nose as needed; ingest 1-3 drops; inhale from cupped hands.

Respiratory Blend [AT]
Black Pepper [ATI]
Rosemary [ATI]
Roman Chamomile [ATI]
Bergamot [ATI]

Energy (low)
Extreme Moringa Energy [I]
Pre-Workout Powder [I]
Nitric Oxide Activator [I]
Vitality-Boosting Blend [ATI]
Peppermint [ATI]

Use supplement products as directed. Apply 1-3 drops of oil to bottoms of feet, under nose, or chest as needed; inhale from cupped hands.

Protocol on pg. 153

Epilepsy
Apply 1-3 drops of oil to back of neck, under nose, or on temples or inhale from cupped hands; ingest 2-4 drops of frankincense daily; use Moringa Super Powder daily.

Frankincense [ATI]
Lavender [ATI]
Vetiver [ATI]
Nourishing Blend [ATI]
Moringa Super Powder [I]

Erectile Dysfunction
Nitric Oxide Activator [ATI]
Cypress [ATI]
Men's Daily Balancing [I]
Sandalwood [ATI]
Ylang Ylang [ATI]

Use nitric oxide activator. Apply 1-3 drops of oil to temples, wrists, and back of neck as needed; inhale from cupped hands.

Estrogen Imbalance
Use aging formula & women's blend daily. Apply 1-3 drops of oil to feet, abdomen, and lower back; inhale from cupped hands; ingest Clary Sage as needed.

Optimal Aging Formula [I]
Women's Daily Balancing [I]
Detoxification Blend [ATI]
Clary Sage [ATI]
Basil [ATI]

Exhaustion
Extreme Moringa Energy [I]
AM Exercise Caps [I]
Ylang Ylang [ATI]
Tangerine [ATI]
Peppermint [ATI]

Use Moringa and caps as needed. Inhale 1-3 drops from cupped hands; apply a couple drops to feet and back; ingest 1-3 drops Ylang Ylang or Tangerine as needed.

Eyes (swollen)
Apply 1-3 drops around the opening of the eye or apply to a cotton ball and place over eye. Do NOT apply into eye.

Geranium [ATI]
Scotch Pine [AT]
Detoxification Blend [ATI]
Patchouli [ATI]
Juniper Berry [ATI]

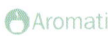 Aromatic 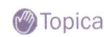 Topical 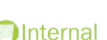 Internal

24

Fainting

Nitric Oxide Activator [I]
Frankincense [A T I]
Respiratory Blend [A T]
Rosemary [A T I]
Eucalyptus [A T I]

Use nitric oxide activator. Inhale 1-3 drops of oil from cupped hands as need.

Fear

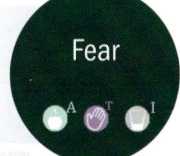

Inhale from cupped hands; apply a couple drops to feet and back of neck.

Stress-Control Blend [A T]
Orange [A T]
Balancing Blend [A T]
Juniper Berry [A T]
Comforting Blend [A T]

Fever

Extreme Moringa Energy [I]
Peppermint [A T I]
Eucalyptus [A T I]
Soothing Blend [A T]
Oregano [A T I]

Use Moringa energy to boost immune system. Apply 1-3 drops of oil to back of neck or chest; ingest 2-4 drops Oregano every 2-4 hours until symptoms subside.

Fibrocystic Breasts

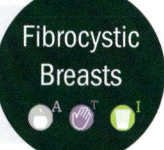

Massage 1-3 drops into breasts as needed; ingest at least twice daily.

Thyme [T I]
Clary Sage [T I]
Sandalwood [T I]
Geranium [T I]
Frankincense [T I]

Fibroids (Uterine)

Optimal Aging Formula [I]
Lemongrass [T I]
Frankincense [T I]
Antioxidant Blend [T I]
Helichrysum [T I]

Use aging formula daily. Apply 1-3 drops of oil to abdomen daily; ingest 1-3 drops.

Fibromyalgia

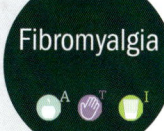

Protocol on pg. 154

Use activator daily. Apply 1-3 drops of oil to affected areas; ingest Frankincense as needed; supplement regularly for long-term support.

Nitric Oxide Activator [I]
Frankincense [A T I]
Wintergreen [A T]
Soothing Blend [A T]
Restorative Blend [A T]

Flu

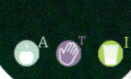

Moringa Super Powder [I]
Immunity-Boosting Blend [A T I]
Respiratory Blend [A T]
Thyme [A T I]
Digestive Support Blend [A T I]

Use Moringa to boost immune system. Apply 1-3 drops of oil to chest or back over lungs; ingest 2-4 drops every 2-3 hours as needed.

Protocol on pg. 154

Focus

Protocol on pg. 143

Use activator daily. Apply 1-3 drops of oil to forehead, temples, back of neck, and behind the ears; inhale from cupped hands as needed.

Nitric Oxide Activator [I]
Vetiver [A T I]
Balancing Blend [A T]
Focusing Blend [A T]
Spearmint [A T I]

Aromatic   Topical   Internal

Food Poisoning

- Detoxification Blend [T][I]
- Digestive Support Blend [T][I]
- Oregano [T][I]
- Protecting Blend [T][I]
- Black Pepper [T][I]

Apply 1-3 drops to stomach and rub clockwise; ingest 2-4 drops every 2-4 hours as needed.

Frozen Shoulder

Use activator as needed. Apply 1-3 drops to affected area. Massage with carrier oil for improved efficacy.

- Nitric Oxide Activator [I]
- Soothing Blend [A][T]
- Cypress [A][T]
- Balsam Fir [A][T][I]
- Restorative Blend [A][T]

Fungal Skin

- Tea Tree [T]
- Atlas Cedarwood [T]
- Skin-Enriching Blend [T]
- Copaiba [T]
- Blue Tansy [T]

Apply 1-3 drops to affected area several times daily.

Gallbladder Issues

Massage 1-3 drops over gallbladder several times daily; ingest 1-3 drops as needed.

- Detoxification Blend [T][I]
- Basil [T][I]
- Weight Control Blend [T][I]
- Helichrysum [T][I]
- Tangerine [T][I]

Gallbladder Stones

- Lemon [T][I]
- Lime [T][I]
- Juniper Berry [T][I]
- Bergamot [T][I]
- Balsam Fir [T][I]

Apply 1-3 drops over gallbladder several times daily; ingest 1-3 drops as needed.

Gas (flatulence)

Protocol on pg. 153

Massage 1-3 drops over stomach; ingest 1-3 drops as needed.

- Fennel [T][I]
- Dill [T][I]
- Digestive Support Blend [T][I]
- Ginger [T][I]
- Tangerine [T][I]

Gastritis

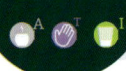

- Moringa Super Powder [T][I]
- Lavender [T][I]
- Ginger [T][I]
- Helichrysum [T][I]
- Coriander [T][I]

Use Moringa to support digestive system. Massage 1-3 drops into stomach area; ingest 1-2 drops diluted in carrier oil inside a veggie cap as needed.

Protocol on pg. 153

Genital Warts

Dilute heavily with a carrier oil and apply 1-3 drops to affected area; ingest 1-3 drops a couple times daily.

- Frankincense [T]
- Patchouli [T]
- Thyme [T]
- Geranium [T]
- Atlas Cedarwood [T]

Aromatic · Topical · Internal

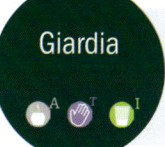

Giardia

Oregano [T I]
Rosemary [T I]
Digestive Support Blend [T I]
Spearmint [T I]
Tea Tree [T I]

Massage 1-3 drops clockwise onto stomach and chest area; ingest 1-3 drops as needed.

Gargle 1-3 drops mixed with water several times daily; ingest 1-3 drops as needed.

Protecting Blend [T I]
Clove [T I]
Tea Tree [T I]
Myrrh [T I]
Atlas Cedarwood [T I]

Gingivitis

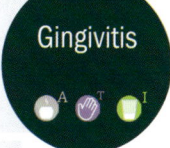

Gluten Sensitivity

Premium Tea [I]
Optimal Aging Formula [I]
Digestive Support Blend [T I]
Lemongrass [T I]
Antioxidant Blend [T I]

Use tea and aging formula daily. Ingest 1-3 drops of oil as needed; rub a few drops onto stomach.

Protocol on pg. 145

Use nitric activator daily. Ingest 1-3 drops of oil twice daily; massage gently into affected joints as needed.

Nitric Oxide Activator [I]
Lemongrass [A T]
Wintergreen [A T]
Spruce [A T]
Soothing Blend [A T]

Gout

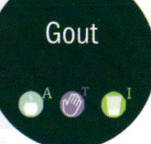

Growing Pains

Moringa Super Powder [I]
Lemongrass [A T I]
Marjoram [A T I]
Soothing Blend [A T]
Restorative Blend [A T]

Use Moringa daily. Massage 1-3 drops of oil into affected area as needed.

Use Moringa to strengthen immune system. Apply 1-3 drops of oil to gums; gargle a few drops in water as needed.

Moringa Super Powder [I]
Clove [T I]
Myrrh [T I]
Protecting Blend [T I]
Tea Tree [T I]

Gum Disease

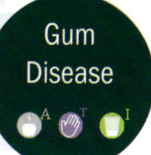

Gums (bleeding)

Helichrysum [T I]
Myrrh [T I]
Clove [T I]
Tea Tree [T I]
Geranium [T I]

Apply 1-3 drops to gums; gargle a couple of drops in water.

Use aging formula daily. Dilute 5 drops of oil in 20 drops of carrier oil, and massage into scalp every night.

Optimal Aging Formula [I]
Rosemary [T]
Nourishing Blend [T I]
Clary Sage [T]
Cypress [T]

Hair Loss

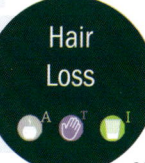

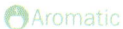 Aromatic   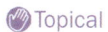 Topical   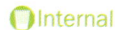 Internal

Ailments

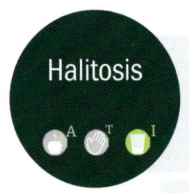

Halitosis
Cinnamon[I]
Protecting Blend[I]
Spearmint[I]
Peppermint[I]
Detoxification Blend[I]

Gargle a few drops mixed with water several times daily or as needed; ingest 1-3 drops Detoxification Blend twice daily.

Hand, Foot & Mouth
Use Moringa energy to boost immune system. Apply 1-3 drops of oil diluted to affected areas; ingest as needed.

Extreme Moringa Energy[I]
Nourishing Blend[T I]
Protecting Blend[T I]
Tea Tree[T I]
Lemongrass[T I]

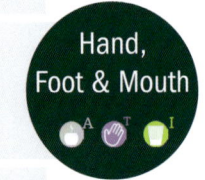

Hangover
Post-Workout Powder[I]
Extreme Moringa Energy[I]
Peppermint[A T I]
Digestive Support Blend[A T I]
Detoxification Blend[A T I]

Drink powder and Moringa energy. Add 4-6 drops of oil to warm bath; massage into back of neck and over liver; ingest 2-4 drops as needed.

Hay Fever
Protocol on pg. 144

Use Moringa to boost immune response. Apply 1-3 drops of oil to under nose or chest as needed; use Lavender under the tongue; inhale from cupped hands.

Moringa Super Powder[I]
Respiration Blend[A T]
Lavender[A T I]
Purifying Blend[A T]
Respiratory Blend[A T]

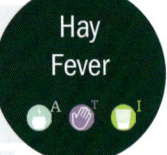

Head Lice
Tea Tree[T]
Atlas Cedarwood[T]
Purifying Blend[T]
Rosemary[T]
Eucalyptus[T]

Dilute 1-3 drops and apply to entire scalp, shampoo, and rinse 30 minutes later. Repeat daily for several days.

Headache
Use nitric oxide activator at the onset of a headache. Massage 1-3 drops of oil into forehead, temples, and back of neck; inhale from cupped hands.

Nitric Oxide Activator[I]
Peppermint[A T I]
Frankincense[A T I]
Soothing Blend[A T]
Spearmint[A T I]

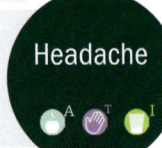

Hearing Issues
Frankincense[T]
Helichrysum[T]
Tea Tree[T]
Basil[T]
Patchouli[T]

Apply 1-3 drops to temples and around the opening of the ear; apply to a cotton ball and place over ear for 15 minutes. Do NOT apply into ear.

Heart Disease
Use nitric oxide activator and Moringa daily. Apply 1-3 drops over chest; ingest 1-3 drops as a daily supplement.

Nitric Oxide Activator[I]
Moringa Super Powder[I]
Marjoram[T I]
Geranium[T I]
Helichrysum[T I]

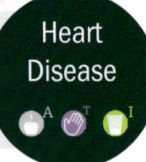

Aromatic Topical Internal

Ailment	Oils	Instructions
Heartburn 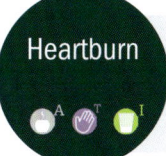	Digestive Support Blend ᵀᴵ Peppermint ᵀᴵ Ginger ᵀᴵ Slimming Blend ᵀᴵ Fennel ᵀᴵ	Massage 1-3 drops into abdomen; ingest 1-3 drops as needed. *Protocol on pg. 154*
Heat Exhaustion 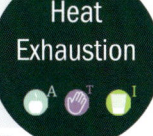	Hydration Powder ᴵ Peppermint ᴬᵀᴵ Scotch Pine ᴬᵀ Lemon ᴬᵀᴵ Grapefruit ᴬᵀᴵ	Use hydration powder. Apply 1-3 drops of oil to forehead, back of neck, and bottom of feet; add lemon or peppermint to mineral water and sip slowly.
Heatstroke	Hydration Powder ᴵ Fennel ᴬᵀᴵ Spearmint ᴬᵀᴵ Peppermint ᴬᵀᴵ Detoxification Blend ᴬᵀᴵ	Use hydration powder. Apply 1-3 drops of oil to forehead, temples, back of neck, and chest; ingest 1-3 drops as needed.
Heavy Metal Detox 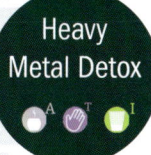	Premium Tea ᴵ Frankincense ᵀᴵ Nourishing Blend ᵀᴵ Detoxification Blend ᵀᴵ Coriander ᵀᴵ	Use tea daily. Ingest 2-4 drops of oil two times daily; massage 2-4 drops into bottoms of feet.
Hematoma	Nitric Oxide Activator ᴵ Cypress ᵀ Massage Blend ᵀ Geranium ᵀᴵ Helichrysum ᵀᴵ	Use activator as directed. Apply 1-3 drops of oil to affected areas 2 to 3 times daily or as needed.
Hemorrhoids 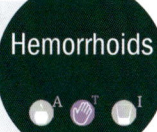	Helichrysum ᵀ Cypress ᵀ Geranium ᵀ Myrrh ᵀ Balsam Fir ᵀ	Dilute 2-4 drops with carrier oil and apply directly to affected areas daily or as needed.
Hepatitis	Moringa Super Powder ᵀᴵ Geranium ᵀᴵ Myrrh ᵀᴵ Detoxification Blend ᵀᴵ Helichrysum ᵀᴵ	Use Moringa daily. Ingest 1-3 drops of oil; use topically with a warm compress over the liver area.
Hernia (hiatal) 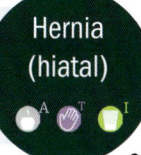	Nitric Oxide Activator ᴵ Helichrysum ᵀ Cypress ᵀ Geranium ᵀ Basil ᵀ	Use nitric oxide activator for several days. Massage 1-3 drops of oil into affected area as needed.

Aromatic   Topical   Internal

Ailments

Herniated Disc	Nitric Oxide Activator [I] Premium Tea [I] Moringa Super Powder [I] Soothing Blend [A T] Restorative Blend [A T]	Use activator, Moringa, and tea to ease inflammation. Massage 1-3 drops of oil into affected area as needed.

	Use Moringa to boost immune system. Ingest 1-3 drops of oil; use topically with a warm compress over the kidneys and left side of throat daily.	Moringa Super Powder [I] Patchouli [T I] Sandalwood [T I] Oregano [T I] Immunity-Boosting Blend [T I]	Herpes Simplex

Hiccups	Nitric Oxide Activator [I] Lemon [A T I] Comforting Blend [A T] Stress Control Blend [A T] Myrtle [A T I]	Use nitric oxide activator. Inhale 1-3 drops of oil from cupped hands; massage into chest and stomach area as needed.

Protocol on pg. 143	Use Moringa energy to boost immune system. Apply 1-3 drops of oil to bottoms of feet; ingest 1-3 drops twice daily; inhale from cupped hands for emotional support.	Extreme Moringa Energy [I] Oregano [A T I] Frankincense [A T I] Black Pepper [A T I] Immunity-Boosting Blend [A T I]	HIV 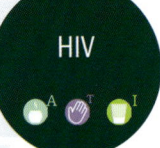

Hives	Nitric Oxide Activator [I] Tea Tree [T I] Frankincense [T I] Lavender [T I] Skin-Enriching Blend [T]	Use nitric oxide activator. Apply 1-3 drops of oil to affected area; ingest 2-4 drops twice daily as needed.

	Use hydration powder throughout the day. Gargle 1-3 drops of water in water as needed; rub a couple drops onto outside of throat.	Hydration Powder [I] Lemon [T I] Myrrh [T I] Protecting Blend [T I] Lavender [T I]	Hoarse Voice 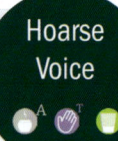

Hormone Imbalance	Optimal Aging Formula [I] Woman's/Men's Balancing [I] Clary Sage [A T I] Monthly Blend [A T] Ylang Ylang [A T I]	Use aging formula daily. Massage 1-3 drops of oil into abdomen, temples, and bottoms of feet; ingest as needed; inhale from cupped hands.

Protocol on pg. 157	Use aging formula daily. Massage 1-3 drops of oil into chest, neck, and face as needed; ingest Clary Sage and Ylang Ylang as needed.	Optimal Aging Formula [I] Monthly Blend [A T] Peppermint [A T I] Clary Sage [A T I] Ylang Ylang [A T I]	Hot Flashes 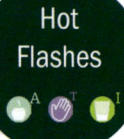

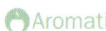 Aromatic 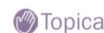 Topical   Internal

Hyperactivity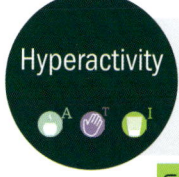

- Daily Tea [I]
- Atlas Cedarwood [A T I]
- Balancing Blend [A T]
- Vetiver [A T I]
- Stress Control Blend [A T]

Use tea for calming. Apply 1-3 drops of oil on back of neck and bottoms of feet; inhale from cupped hands.

Protocol on pg. 161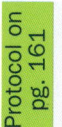

Use tea for calming. Apply 1-2 drops of oil behind ears; inhale from cupped hands.

- Daily Tea [I]
- Balancing Blend [A T]
- Orange [A T I]
- Focusing Blend [A T]
- Myrtle [A T I]

Hypertension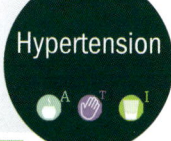

Hyperthyroid (Grave's)

- Optimal Aging Formula [I]
- Myrrh [T I]
- Frankincense [T I]
- Detoxification Blend [T I]
- Rosemary [T I]

Use aging formula daily. Apply 1-3 drops over thyroid several times daily. Ingest 1-3 drops a few times daily or as needed.

Protocol on pg. 162

Use workout powder for blood sugar. Apply 1-3 drops of oil to chest and inside of wrists; ingest 1-3 drops a few times daily or as needed.

- During Workout Powder [I]
- Weight Control Blend [T I]
- Cinnamon [T I]
- Coriander [T I]
- Detoxification Blend [T I]

Hypoglycemia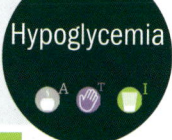

Hypothyroid (Hashimoto's)

- Nitric Oxide Activator [I]
- Moringa Super Powder [I]
- Clove [T I]
- Peppermint [T I]
- Lemongrass [T I]

Use Moringa and activator daily. Apply 1-3 drops over thyroid several times daily; ingest 1-3 drops a few times daily or as needed.

Protocol on pg. 163

Protocol on pg. 155

Use Moringa energy as directed. Apply 2-4 drops of oil to bottoms of feet; ingest as needed; inhale from cupped hands as needed.

- Extreme Moringa Energy [I]
- Protecting Blend [A T I]
- Oregano [A T I]
- Tea Tree [A T I]
- Black Pepper [A T I]

Immune Boost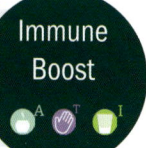

Indigestion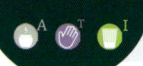

- Digestive Supportive Blend [T I]
- Black Pepper [T I]
- Weight Control Blend [T I]
- Ginger [T I]
- Orange [T I]

Massage 1-3 drops into stomach area clockwise, or take with water or in a capsule.

Protocol on pg. 154

Dilute with carrier oil and apply 1-3 drops to stomach area and chest as needed.

- Fennel [T]
- Digestive Support Blend [T]
- Coriander [T]
- Ginger [T]
- Lavender [T]

Infant Reflux

Aliments

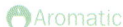 Aromatic 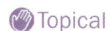 Topical 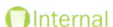 Internal

31

Ailments

Infected Wounds
Myrrh [T]
Helichrysum [T]
Tea Tree [T]
Frankincense [T]
Purifying Blend [T]

Apply 1-3 drops to affected areas 2 to 3 times daily as needed.

Protocol on pg. 155
Use aging formula and activator daily. Apply 1-3 drops of oil to abdomen daily; ingest 1-3 drops as needed; also diffuse several drops daily.

Optimal Aging Formula [I]
Nitric Oxide Activator [I]
Clary Sage [A T I]
Nourishing Blend [A T I]
Women's/Men's Balancing [I]

Infertility
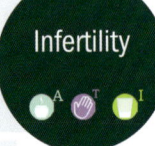

Inflammation
Moringa Super Powder [I]
Nitric Oxide Activator [I]
Soothing Blend [A T]
Frankincense [A T I]
Copaiba [A T I]

Use Moringa and activator. Apply 1-3 drops of oil to affected areas as needed. For systemic inflammation, ingest 2-4 drops twice daily.

Protocol on pg. 155
Massage 1-3 drops into stomach; take a few drops internally as needed.

Digestive Support Blend [T I]
Spearmint [T I]
Detoxification Blend [T I]
Ginger [T I]
Lavender [T I]

Inflammatory Bowls
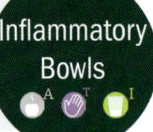

Ingrown Toenail
Tea Tree [T]
Ylang Ylang [T]
Nourishing Blend [T]
Detoxification Blend [T]
Clove [T]

Apply 1-3 drops to affected toenail as needed.

Apply a drop or two to insect bites hourly or as needed.

Lavender [T]
Purifying Blend [T]
Roman Chamomile [T]
Tea Tree [T]
Sandalwood [T]

Insect Bites
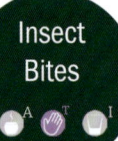

Insomnia
Premium Tea [I]
Comforting Blend [A T]
Atlas Cedarwood [A T I]
Stress Control Blend [A T]
Vetiver [A T I]

Use tea before bedtime. Apply 1-3 drops of oil to forehead, temples, base of skull, and behind the ears; use in a diffuser.

Protocol on pg. 160

Protocol on pg. 152
Use Moringa and activator daily. Apply 1-3 drops of oil to bottoms of feet; take a few drops internally as needed.

Moringa Super Powder [I]
Nitric Oxide Activator [I]
Coriander [T I]
Oregano [T I]
Weight Control Blend [T I]

Insulin Imbalance

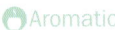 Aromatic   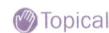 Topical   Internal

Irritable Bowels

Digestive Support Blend [T I]
Ginger [T I]
Peppermint [T I]
Lavender [T I]
Vetiver [T I]

Apply 1-3 drops to stomach as needed; take internally with water or in a capsule.

Protocol on pg. 155

Itchy Skin

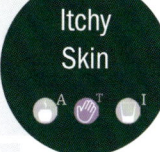

Protocol on pg. 153

Use Moringa-enhanced skincare products. Apply 1-3 drops of oil to affected areas as needed. Use with carrier oil or lotion for improved efficacy.

Moringa Skin Products
Skin-Enriching Blend [T]
Atlas Cedarwood [T]
Ylang Ylang [T]
German Chamomile [T]

Jaundice

Detoxification Blend [A T I]
Geranium [A T I]
Rosemary [A T I]
Juniper Berry [A T I]
Cilantro [A T I]

Massage 1-3 drops diluted over the liver; ingest 1-3 drops as needed (for adults); diffuse next to baby's crib.

Jet Lag

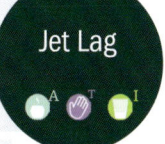

Use Limitless Energy Powder or Moringa energy. Apply 1-3 drops of oil to forehead, temples, back of neck, and chest; inhale from cupped hands as needed.

Limitless Energy Powder [I]
Extreme Moringa Energy [I]
Peppermint [A T I]
Tangerine [A T I]
Antioxidant Blend [A T I]

Jock Itch

Moringa Super Powder [I]
Tea Tree [T I]
Thyme [T I]
Patchouli [T I]
Purifying Blend [T]

Use Moringa to assist with inflammation and irritation. Apply 1-3 drops to affected areas as needed with carrier oil; ingest a few drops as needed.

Joint Pain

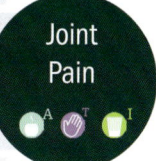

Protocol on pg. 145

Use Moringa and activator daily. Massage 1-3 drops of oil into affected areas as needed.

Moringa Super Powder [I]
Nitric Oxide Activator [I]
Soothing Blend [A T]
Wintergreen [A T]
Lemongrass [A T I]

Kidney Infection

Extreme Moringa Energy [I]
Lemongrass [T I]
Cinnamon [T I]
Juniper Berry [T I]
Cypress [T]

Use Moringa energy to strengthen immune system. Apply 1-3 drops of oil to kidney area a couple times daily; ingest 1-3 drops as needed.

Massage 1-3 drops over kidneys; ingest 1-3 drops as needed.

Lemon [T I]
Lemongrass [T I]
Sandalwood [T I]
Clary Sage [T I]
Wintergreen [T]

Kidney Stones

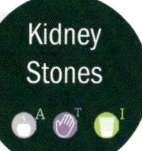

Ailments

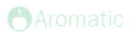 Aromatic   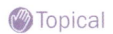 Topical   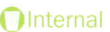 Internal

33

Ailments

Lactose Intolerance
- Digestive Support Blend [TI]
- Coriander [TI]
- Lemongrass [TI]
- Detoxification Blend [TI]
- Frankincense [TI]

Ingest 2-4 drops or massage onto stomach as needed.

Laryngitis
Use Moringa energy to boost immune system. Diffuse oils throughout the day; massage 1-3 drops on outside of throat.
- Extreme Moringa Energy [I]
- Protecting Blend [ATI]
- Myrrh [ATI]
- Lavender [ATI]
- Frankincense [ATI]

Leg Cramps
- Nitric Oxide Activator [I]
- Cypress [ATI]
- Soothing Blend [ATI]
- Restorative Blend [ATI]
- Blue Tansy [ATI]

Use activator as needed. Massage several drops of oil, diluting Blue Tansy to avoid blue staining.

Leukemia
Use Moringa for nutrition support. Ingest 2-4 drops of oil three times daily; massage into bottoms of feet frequently.
- Moringa Super Powder [I]
- Frankincense [ATI]
- Nourishing Blend [ATI]
- Lemongrass [ATI]
- Detoxification Blend [ATI]

Libido (low)
- Nitric Oxide Activator [I]
- Ylang Ylang [ATI]
- Monthly Blend [AT]
- Cinnamon [ATI]
- Juniper Berry [ATI]

Use activator daily. Massage 1-3 drops of oil into abdomen, bottoms of feet, and temples; inhale from cupped hands or diffuse.

Protocol on pg. 156

Lyme Disease
Protocol on pg. 156

Use activator daily. Massage 2-4 drops of oil into lower back a couple times daily as needed, and ingest in a capsule.
- Nitric Oxide Activator [I]
- Clove [ATI]
- Cinnamon [ATI]
- Thyme [ATI]
- Oregano [ATI]

Lupus
- Moringa Super Powder [I]
- Soothing Blend [AT]
- Nourishing Blend [ATI]
- Frankincense [ATI]
- Detoxification Blend [ATI]

Use Moringa for nutritional support. Ingest 2-4 drops of oil twice daily during flair ups; massage with carrier oil onto inflamed areas.

Protocol on pg. 156

Measles
Use Moringa energy to boost immune system. Dab a few drops of oil onto spots several times daily; add several drops to bath and soak for 30 minutes.
- Extreme Moringa Energy [I]
- Eucalyptus [TI]
- Tea Tree [TI]
- Lavender [TI]
- Protecting Blend [TI]

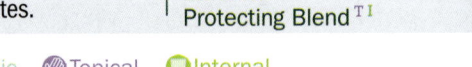

Melanoma
Optimal Aging Formula [I]
Sandalwood [T I]
Nourishing Blend [T I]
Frankincense [T I]
Atlas Cedarwood [T I]

Use aging formula as directed. Apply 1-3 drops of oil to affected areas; ingest 2-4 drops twice daily.

Memory Loss
Use activator and aging formula. Massage 1-3 drops of oil into forehead, temples, and back of neck; inhale from cupped hands.

Nitric Oxide Activator [I]
Optimal Aging Formula [I]
Rosemary [A T I]
Peppermint [A T I]
Focusing Blend [A T]

Meningitis
Extreme Moringa Energy [I]
Lemongrass [T I]
Protecting Blend [T I]
Tea Tree [T I]
Basil [T I]

Use Moringa energy to boost immune system. Ingest 2-4 drops twice daily; massage 2-4 drops into back of neck with carrier oil daily.

Menopause
Protocol on pg. 157

Use Moringa daily. Apply a few drops of oil topically to abdomen, bottoms of feet, and back of neck daily; ingest Clary Sage and Balsam Fir as needed.

Moringa Super Powder [I]
Clary Sage [A T I]
Balsam Fir [A T I]
Women's Balancing Blend [I]
Monthly Blend [A T]

Menstrual Bleeding
Helichrysum [T I]
Geranium [T I]
Clary Sage [T I]
Monthly Blend [T I]
Detoxification Blend [T I]

Massage 2-4 drops into abdomen, lower back, and shoulders; apply to a warm compress over uterus area; ingest 2-4 drops as needed.

Menstrual Pain
Protocol on pg. 157

Use aging formula. Massage 1-3 drops of oil into abdomen, lower back, and shoulders; apply to a warm compress over uterus area; ingest 2-4 drops as needed.

Optimal Aging Formula [I]
Clary Sage [A T I]
Monthly Blend [A T]
Marjoram [A T I]
Frankincense [A T I]

Mental Fatigue
Limitless Energy Powder [I]
Peppermint [A T I]
Rosemary [A T I]
Bergamot [A T I]
Scotch Pine [A T]

Use energy mix as needed. Massage 1-3 drops of oil into forehead, temples, back of neck, and bottoms of feet; inhale from cupped hands as needed.

Migraine
Use the aging formula to decrease inflammation. Apply 1-3 drops of oil to forehead, temples, and base of skull; inhale from cupped hands as needed.

Optimal Aging Formula [I]
Peppermint [A T I]
Soothing Blend [A T]
Frankincense [A T I]
Lavender [A T I]

Ailments

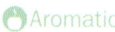 Aromatic   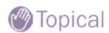 Topical   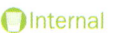 Internal

35

Ailments

Mold & Mildew
Protecting Blend [AT]
Tea Tree [AT]
Oregano [AT]
Spruce [AT]
Purifying Blend [AT]

Diffuse into the air where mold is present several times daily until no longer needed. Mix 20 drops with 4 oz water and apply to area of concern.

Moles
Apply a drop to mole 2-3 times daily until it disappears. Avoid surrounding skin when using Oregano.

Oregano [T]
Frankincense [T]
Skin-Enriching Blend [T]
Nourishing Blend [T]
Sandalwood [T]

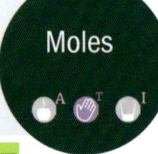

Mononucleosis
Extreme Moringa Energy [I]
Thyme [ATI]
Black Pepper [ATI]
Oregano [ATI]
Protecting Blend [ATI]

Use Moringa energy to boost immune system and energy levels. Ingest 1-3 drops of oil twice a day; apply to bottoms of feet; diffuse several drops.

Protocol on pg. 157

Mood Swings
Use caps to stabilize mood. Inhale 1-3 drops of oil from cupped hands; apply a few drops to forehead, temples, back of neck, and bottoms of feet.

PM Craving Control Caps [I]
Patchouli [AT]
Comforting Blend [AT]
Balancing Blend [AT]
Stress Control Blend [AT]

Morning Sickness
Ginger [ATI]
Peppermint [ATI]
Digestive Support Blend [ATI]
Fennel [ATI]
Coriander [ATI]

Apply 1-3 drops behind ears and over navel hourly; inhale from cupped hands; ingest 1-3 drops as needed.

Protocol on pg. 158

Motion Sickness
Apply 1-3 drops behind the ears and over navel; inhale from cupped hands; or take internally.

Peppermint [ATI]
Digestive Support Blend [ATI]
Ginger [ATI]
Balancing Blend [AT]
Basil [ATI]

Mouth Ulcers
Extreme Moringa Energy [I]
Protecting Blend [TI]
Clove [TI]
Myrrh [TI]
Tea Tree [TI]

Use Moringa energy to boost immune system. Gargle 1-3 drops of oil mixed with water several times daily; apply to gums; ingest as needed.

Muscle Injury
Protocol on pg. 158

Use activator during injury. Massage 1-3 drops of oil into affected muscles as needed.

Nitric Oxide Activator [I]
Marjoram [TI]
Helichrysum [TI]
Basil [TI]
Massage Blend [T]

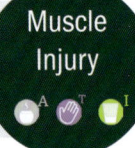

36

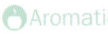 Aromatic   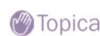 Topical   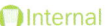 Internal

Muscle Pain
A T I

Moringa Super Powder [I]
Soothing Blend [A T]
Copaiba [A T I]
Massage Blend [A T]
Restorative Blend [A T]

Use Moringa daily. Massage 1-3 drops of oil into affected muscles as needed; inhale from cupped hands or diffuse as well.

Protocol on pg. 158

Muscle Spasms
A T I

Use activator as needed. Massage 1-3 drops of oil into affected muscles; inhale from cupped hands; put a drop under tongue.

Nitric Oxide Activator [I]
Black Pepper [A T I]
Basil [A T I]
Coriander [A T I]
Lemongrass [A T I]

Muscle Stiffness
A T I

Nitric Oxide Activator [I]
Massage Blend [T I]
Soothing Blend [T I]
Lemongrass [T I]
Scotch Pine [T I]

Use activator as needed. Massage 1-3 of oils into stiff muscles as needed.

Protocol on pg. 158

Nasal Congestion
A T I

Apply 1-3 drops over bridge of nose, under nose, and rub over sinuses. Use carrier oil if desired.

Respiratory Blend [A T]
Balsam Fir [A T I]
Respiration Blend [A T]
Eucalyptus [A T I]
Peppermint [A T I]

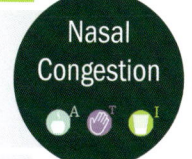

Nasal Polyps
A T I

Rosemary [A T]
Frankincense [A T]
Respiratory Blend [A T]
Sandalwood [A T]
Geranium [A T]

Apply 1-3 drops over bridge of nose and under nose; ingest 1-3 drops twice daily.

Nausea
A T I

Use tea when available. Apply 1-3 drops of oil behind ears and over navel hourly; ingest under the tongue; inhale from cupped hands.

Daily Tea [I]
Ginger [A T I]
Digestive Support Blend [A T I]
Peppermint [A T I]
Detoxification Blend [A T I]

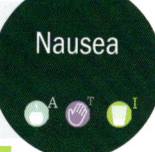

Neck Pain
A T I

Optimal Aging Formula [I]
Nitric Oxide Activator [I]
Soothing Blend [A T]
Wintergreen [A T]
Lemongrass [A T]

Use aging formula with activator. Massage 1-3 drops of oil onto neck several times daily. Blend with carrier oil to improve efficacy.

Protocol on pg. 146

Nervous Fatigue
A T I

Use activator and capsules. Inhale oils from cupped hands; apply 1-3 drops to temples, behind ears, and on back of neck as needed.

Nitric Oxide Activator [I]
Extreme Moringa Caps [I]
Basil [A T I]
Tangerine [A T I]
Rosemary [A T I]

Ailments

🟢 Aromatic 🟣 Topical ⚪ Internal

Ailments

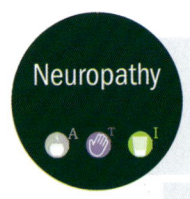

Neuropathy
_{A T I}

Nitric Oxide Activator[I]
Cypress[T I]
Massage Blend[T I]
Vetiver[T I]
Soothing Blend[T I]

Use activator daily. Apply 1-3 drops of oil to affected areas several times daily; ingest 1-3 drops as needed.

Night Sweats
_{A T I}

Use powder to restore the body. Apply 1-3 drops of oil to abdomen and back of neck before sleeping; ingest as needed.

Post-Workout Powder[I]
Detoxification Blend[T I]
Nourishing Blend[I]
Lime[T I]
Peppermint[T I]

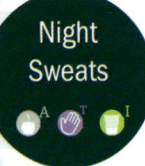

Nightmares
_{A T I}

Juniper Berry[A T I]
Roman Chamomile[A T I]
Lavender[A T I]
Stress Control Blend[A T]
Comforting Blend[A T]

Apply 1-3 drops to abdomen and back of neck before sleeping; ingest as needed.

Nosebleed
_{T I}

Use hydration powder and activator for restorative benefits. Apply 1-3 drops of oil to the bridge and sides of nose and back of neck as needed.

Hydration Powder[I]
Nitric Oxide Activator[I]
Helichrysum[T]
Geranium[T]
Myrrh[T]

Odors
_{A T I}

Premium Tea[I]
Purifying Blend[A T]
Tea Tree[A T I]
Atlas Cedarwood[A T I]
Balsam Fir[A T I]

Use tea daily. Use oils in a diffuser or spray bottle for external odors. Ingest 2-3 drops twice daily for body odors.

Osteoarthritis
_{A T I}

Use aging blend and Moringa for inflammatory support. Massage 1-3 drops of oil into affected areas as often as needed; inhale from cupped hands.

Optimal Aging Blend[I]
Moringa Super Powder[I]
Soothing Blend[A T]
Lemongrass[A T]
Wintergreen[A T]

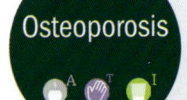

Osteoporosis
_{A T I}

Optimal Aging Blend[I]
Moringa Super Powder[I]
Lemongrass[T I]
Clove[T I]
Nourishing Blend[T I]

Use aging blend and Moringa daily. Massage 1-3 drops onto spine and affected areas daily; take Lemongrass or Nourishing Blend internally.

Ovarian Cysts
_{A T I}

Blend 1-3 drops with carrier oil and soak tampon, insert overnight; or apply warm compress over the stomach; take internally.

Frankincense[T I]
Clary Sage[T I]
Basil[T I]
Sandalwood[T I]
Nourishing Blend[T I]

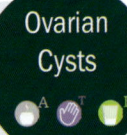

○ Aromatic   ○ Topical   ○ Internal

Overeating
A T I

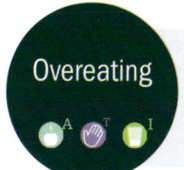

Extreme Moringa Caps [I]
Daily Tea [I]
Slimming Blend [A T I]
Weight Control Blend [A T I]
Peppermint [A T I]

Use capsules and tea daily. Apply 1-3 drops of oil to stomach; take a few drops internally; inhale from cupped hands or diffuse throughout the day.

Protocol on pg. 163

Use aging formula as directed. Apply 1-3 drops of oil over chest as needed; inhale from cupped hands or diffuse.

Optimal Aging Formula [I]
Lavender [A T I]
Geranium [A T I]
Ylang Ylang [A T I]
Orange [A T I]

Palpitations
A T I

Pancreatitis
A T I

Optimal Aging Formula [I]
Detoxification Blend [T I]
Marjoram [T I]
Lemon [T I]
Rosemary [T I]

Use aging formula. Ingest 1-3 drops of oil several times weekly; massage 1-3 drops on abdomen as needed.

Protocol on pg. 152

Use tea for several days. Ingest 2-4 drops of oil; apply in a warm compress over intestinal area 2 to 3 times daily.

Premium Tea [I]
Detoxification Blend [T I]
Oregano [T I]
Thyme [T I]
Immunity-Boosting Blend [T I]

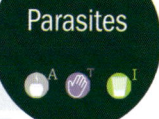

Parasites
A T I

Pink Eye/ Conjunctivitis
A T I

Tea Tree [T]
Rosemary [T]
Atlas Cedarwood [T]
Clary Sage [T]
Purifying Blend [T]

Apply a drop or two around (but not in) eyes. Rub in with carrier oil and be cautious around the eyes.

Apply 1-3 drops to wart several times daily.

Oregano [T]
Nourishing Blend [T]
Frankincense [T]
Antioxidant Blend [T]

Plantar Warts
A T I

Pneumonia
A T I

Extreme Moringa Energy [I]
Protecting Blend [A T I]
Bergamot [A T I]
Thyme [A T I]
Roman Chamomile [A T I]

Use Moringa energy to boost immune system. Apply 1-3 drops to chest and neck area 3 to 5 times daily and gargle hourly; inhale from cupped hands as needed.

Protocol on pg. 147

Use a Moringa-enhanced lotion. Apply 1-3 drops of oil to affected area with carrier oil several times daily or as needed.

Moringa Skincare Products [T]
Lavender [T]
Frankincense [T]
Sandalwood [T]
Geranium [T]

Poison Ivy/Oak
A T I

Ailments

🌿 Aromatic   ✋ Topical   💊 Internal

39

Ailments

PTSD
- Nitric Oxide Activator [I]
- Comforting Blend [A T]
- Restorative Blend [A T]
- Ylang Ylang [A T]
- Helichrysum [A T]

Use activator daily. Apply 1-3 drops of oil to forehead, temples, back of neck, chest, and bottoms of feet; inhale from cupped hands as needed.

Protocol on pg. 157
Use Moringa for nutritional support. Add 1-3 drops of oil to warm bath; apply to abdomen; inhale from cupped hands; ingest Clary Sage and Geranium as needed.

PMS
- Moringa Super Powder [I]
- Monthly Blend [A T]
- Women's Balancing Blend [A T]
- Clary Sage [A T I]
- Geranium [A T I]

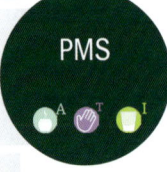

Prostate Issues
- Optimal Aging Formula [I]
- Sandalwood [A T I]
- Frankincense [A T I]
- Nourishing Blend [A T I]
- Men's Balancing Blend [I]

Use aging formula and Men's Balancing Blend daily. Apply oils to the insides of thighs and bottoms of feet morning and night.

Protocol on pg. 159
Use aging formula and Moringa daily. Apply 1-3 drops of oil to affected area a couple times daily with carrier oil; ingest 1-3 drops daily.

Psoriasis
- Optimal Aging Formula [I]
- Moringa Super Powder [I]
- Skin-Enriching Blend [A T]
- Tea Tree [A T I]
- Roman Chamomile [A T I]

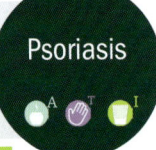

Rashes
- Moringa Skincare Products [T]
- Skin-Enriching Blend [T]
- Roman Chamomile [T I]
- Tea Tree [T I]
- Lavender [T I]

Use a Moringa-enhanced lotion. Dilute 1-3 drops of oil with a carrier oil and apply to affected area as needed. Use a drop of lavender under the tongue for itching.

Protocol on pg. 153
Use activator as directed. Apply 1-3 drops of oil to chest, neck, under nose, and on bridge of nose; inhale from cupped hands or diffuse several drops.

Respiratory Issues
- Nitric Oxide Activator [I]
- Respiratory Blend [A T]
- Eucalyptus [A T I]
- Respiration Blend [A T]
- Scotch Pine [A T]

Restless Leg Syndrome
- Nitric Oxide Activator [I]
- Cypress [A T]
- Massage Blend [A T]
- Stress Control Blend [A T]
- Orange [A T I]

Use activator daily. Massage 1-3 drops of oil onto legs before sleeping; inhale from cupped hands as needed.

Use tea for calming. Inhale oils from cupped hands; apply 1-3 drops to bottoms of feet and back of neck as needed.

Restlessness
- Premium Tea [I]
- Balancing Blend [A T]
- Lavender [A T I]
- Comforting Blend [A T]
- Vetiver [A T I]

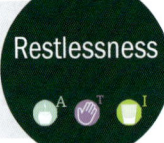

Aromatic | Topical | Internal

Rheumatic Fever
A T I

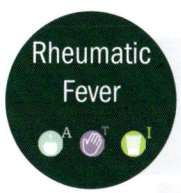

Extreme Moringa Energy [I]
Peppermint [A T I]
Wintergreen [A T]
Protecting Blend [A T I]
Oregano [A T I]

Use Moringa energy to boost immune system. Apply 1-3 drops of oil to bottoms of feet; ingest 1-3 drops twice daily; gargle a few drops mixed with water as needed.

Use activator during symptoms. Inhale 1-3 drops of oil from cupped hands several times daily; apply a couple drops to forehead and bridge of nose; ingest 1-2 drops.

Nitric Oxide Activator [I]
Respiratory Blend [A T]
Tea Tree [A T I]
Peppermint [A T I]
Oregano [A T I]

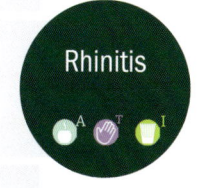

Rhinitis
A T I

Ringworm
A T I

Tea Tree [T I]
Skin-Enriching Blend [T]
Purifying Blend [T]
Thyme [T I]
Lemongrass [T I]

Apply 1-3 drops to affected area 3-4 times daily; ingest a few drops 2-3 times daily for several days.

Rub a couple drops over scarred area twice daily.

Skin-Enriching Blend [T]
Sandalwood [T]
Frankincense [T]
Myrrh [T]
Helichrysum [T]

Scarring
A T

Sciatica
A T I

Optimal Aging Formula [I]
Nitric Oxide Activator [I]
Vetiver [T I]
Helichrysum [T I]
Soothing Blend [T]

Use aging formula and activator daily. Massage 1-3 drops of oil into affected area a couple times daily.

Protocol on pg. 146

Use activator daily. Apply 1-3 drops of oil to back of neck and bottoms of feet; inhale from cupped hands as needed; ingest 1-3 drops twice daily.

Nitric Oxide Activator [I]
Frankincense [A T I]
Balancing Blend [A T]
Sandalwood [A T I]
Focusing Blend [A T]

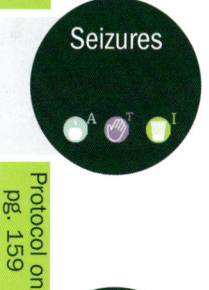

Seizures
A T I

Shingles
A T I

Optimal Aging Formula [I]
Black Pepper [T I]
Tea Tree [T I]
Frankincense [T I]
Geranium [T I]

Use aging formula during symptoms. Apply 1-3 drops to affected area, on back of neck, and along the spine as needed; take 2-4 drops twice daily.

Protocol on pg. 159

Apply 1-3 drops on temples, under nose, and on back of neck as needed; inhale from cupped hands.

AM Exercise Caps [I]
Balancing Blend [A T]
Helichrysum [A T I]
Stress Control Blend [A T]
Tangerine [A T I]

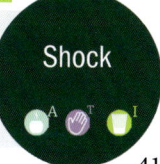

Shock
A T I

Ailments

🟢 Aromatic   🟣 Topical   🟢 Internal

Ailments

Sinus Infection
- Extreme Moringa Energy [I]
- Tea Tree [A T I]
- Black Pepper [A T I]
- Oregano [A T I]
- Respiratory Blend [A T]

Use Moringa energy to boost immune system. Ingest 2-4 drops a few times a day during symptoms; rub 1-3 drops over sinuses and bridge of nose.

Protocol on pg. 159

Skin Ulcers
Use a Moringa-enhanced serum. Apply 1-3 drops to affected area a couple times daily. Dilute if necessary.

- Moringa Skin Products [T]
- Myrrh [T]
- Skin-Enriching Blend [T]
- Sandalwood [T]
- Geranium [T]

Smoking Addiction
- PM Craving Control Caps [I]
- Black Pepper [A T I]
- Grapefruit [A T I]
- Detoxification Blend [A T I]
- Antioxidant Blend [A T I]

Use caps as directed. Ingest 2-4 drops daily; apply Black Pepper to big toe; inhale from cupped hands as needed when experiencing cravings.

Protocol on pg. 160

Snoring
Protocol on pg. 161

Use activator to increase oxygen flow. Apply 1-3 drops of oil to chest and under nose; use in a diffuser beside bed at night.

- Nitric Oxide Activator [I]
- Respiration Blend [A T]
- Respiratory Blend [A T]
- Eucalyptus [A T I]
- Spruce [A T]

Sore Throat
- Extreme Moringa Energy [I]
- Protecting Blend [T I]
- Lavender [T I]
- Lemon [T I]
- Oregano [T I]

Use Moringa energy to boost immune system. Gargle 1-3 drops of oil mixed with water, then swallow; apply to throat and neck, diluting with carrier oil as needed.

Protocol on pg. 161

Sprains
Use aging formula to ease inflammation. Gently apply 1-3 drops of oil to affected area as needed.

- Optimal Aging Formula [I]
- Soothing Blend [T]
- Helichrysum [T]
- Wintergreen [T]
- Massage Blend [T]

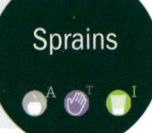

Stomachache
- Ginger [T I]
- Digestive Support Blend [T I]
- Peppermint [T I]
- Orange [T I]
- Roman Chamomile [T I]

Apply 1-3 drops to stomach area as needed; ingest 1-3 drops as needed.

Protocol on pg. 153

Stretch Marks
Use Moringa-enhanced skincare. Apply 1-3 drops of oil to affected areas a couple times daily.

- Moringa Skin Products [T]
- Skin-Enriching Blend [T]
- Geranium [T]
- Frankincense [T]
- Myrrh [T]

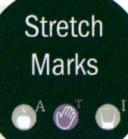

Aromatic • Topical • Internal

Stroke
A T I

Moringa Super Powder [I]
Nitric Oxide Activator [I]
Nourishing Blend [A T I]
Frankincense [A T I]
Cypress [A T]

Use Moringa and activator daily. Apply 1-3 drops on temples, forehead, behind ears, and back of neck; ingest 1-2 times daily.

Protocol on pg. 162

Use Moringa-enhanced skincare. Apply 1-3 drops of oil to affected area hourly or as needed. Blend 2-3 oils, 2-3 drops each with carrier oil for improved results.

Moringa Skin Products [T]
Lavender [T]
Helichrysum [T]
Peppermint [T]
Frankincense [T]

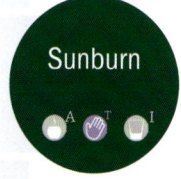

Sunburn
A T

Teething Pain
A T I

Lavender [T]
Clove [T]
Wintergreen [T]
Frankincense [T]
Copaiba [T]

Dilute with carrier oil and gently massage a drop along baby's jawline, reapplying as needed.

Use Moringa to reduce inflammation. Massage 1-3 drops of oil into affected areas 4 to 5 times daily, or as needed.

Extreme Moringa Caps [I]
Lemongrass [A T I]
Marjoram [A T I]
Soothing Blend [A T]
Massage Blend [A T]

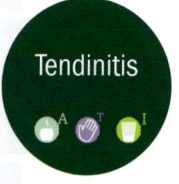

Tendinitis
A T I

Tennis Elbow
A T I

Optimal Aging Formula [I]
Lemongrass [A T I]
Soothing Blend [A T]
Scotch Pine [A T]
Blue Tansy [A T]

Use aging formula to reduce inflammation. Massage 1-3 drops of oil into affected area as needed.

Use Moringa and Men's Balancing Blend daily. Apply 2-4 drops of oil to bottoms of feet twice daily; inhale from cupped hands or diffuse several drops daily.

Moringa Super Powder [I]
Men's Balancing Blend [I]
Patchouli [A T I]
Sandalwood [A T I]
Balancing Blend [A T]

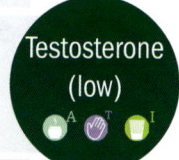

Testosterone (low)
A T I

Thrush
A T I

Lemon [T I]
Orange [T I]
Atlas Cedarwood [T I]
Oregano [T I]
Protecting Blend [T I]

Gargle 1-3 drops mixed with water several times daily; apply topically to lower throat and bottoms of feet; ingest 1-3 drops as needed.

Protocol on pg. 162

Apply 1-3 drops around the opening of the eye or apply to a cotton ball and place over eye. Do NOT apply into eye.

Tea Tree [T]
Purifying Blend [T]
Lavender [T]
Nutmeg [T]
Roman Chamomile [T]

Tick Bites
A T I

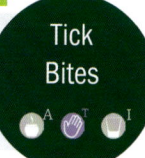

Ailments

🌬️ Aromatic   🟣 Topical   🟢 Internal

Ailments

Tinnitus
Helichrysum [T]
Balancing Blend [T]
Basil [T]
Cypress [T]
Rosemary [T]

Apply 1-2 drops behind ear 2-3 times daily.

Tonsillitis
Use Moringa energy to boost immune system. Gargle 1-3 drops of oil mixed with water or ingest; apply diluted to throat several times daily.

Extreme Moringa Energy [I]
Protecting Blend [T I]
Tea Tree [T I]
Oregano [T I]
Black Pepper [T I]

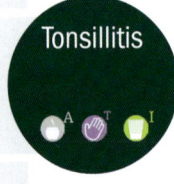

Toothache
Clove [T I]
Protecting Blend [T I]
Tea Tree [T I]
Helichrysum [T I]
Wintergreen [T]

Apply a drop to gums or ingest by adding to water, gargling, and swallowing daily, or as needed.

Trauma (emotional)
Use Moringa for healthy mood. Apply 2-4 drops of oil to forehead, temples, back of neck, and chest; inhale from cupped hands as needed.

Moringa Super Powder [I]
Stress Control Blend [A T]
Balancing Blend [A T]
Comforting Blend [A T]
Helichrysum [A T]

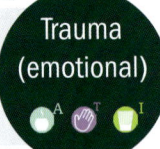

Ulcers (stomach)
Detoxification Blend [T I]
Lemongrass [T I]
Myrrh [T I]
Frankincense [T I]
Geranium [T I]

Ingest 1-3 drops at least once daily; massage gently into abdomen as needed.

Urinary Tract Infection
Use Moringa to boost immune system. Massage 1-3 drops of oil over bladder and on bottoms of the feet; ingest as needed.

Extreme Moringa Caps [I]
Cypress [T]
Juniper Berry [T I]
Basil [T I]
Lemongrass [T I]

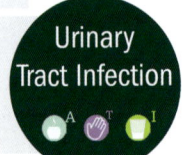

Varicose Veins
Nitric Oxide Activator [I]
Cypress [T]
Helichrysum [T]
Balsam Fir [T]
Detoxification Blend [T]

Use activator daily. Massage 1-3 drops of oil into affected area several times daily.

Vision Loss
Use Moringa and activator daily. Apply 1-3 drops of oil around the opening of eyes or apply to a cotton ball and place over eye. Do NOT apply into eye.

Moringa Super Powder [I]
Nitric Oxide Activator [I]
Clary Sage [T I]
Nourishing Blend [T I]
Helichrysum [T I]

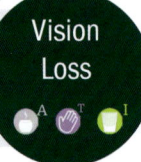

Aromatic   Topical   Internal

Vomiting
[A T I]

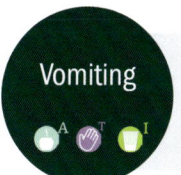

- Digestive Support Blend [A T I]
- Peppermint [A T I]
- Ginger [A T I]
- Bergamot [A T I]
- Roman Chamomile [A T I]

Apply 1-3 drops to stomach area as needed; inhale from cupped hands.

Warts
[A T I]

Apply a drop directly to wart several times daily until the wart disappears. Avoid the surrounding skin with Oregano.

- Oregano [T]
- Frankincense [T]
- Thyme [T]
- Skin-Enriching Blend [T]

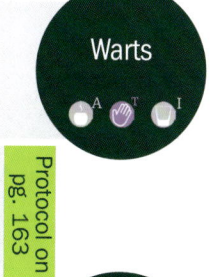

Weight Loss
[A T I]

- PM Craving Control Caps [I]
- Advanced Thermogenic Caps [I]
- All Workout Powders [I]
- Slimming Blend [A T I]
- Weight Control Blend [A T I]

Use caps and workout powders daily. Add 1-3 drops of oil to water to manage cravings and encourage metabolism. Inhale from cupped hands to satisfy cravings.

Protocol on pg. 163

Whiplash
[A T I]

Use activator to encourage circulation. Massage 1-3 drops of oil into affected area as needed. Use with carrier oil to improve efficacy.

- Nitric Oxide Activator [I]
- Soothing Blend [A T]
- Balsam Fir [A T]
- Lemongrass [A T]
- Patchouli [A T]

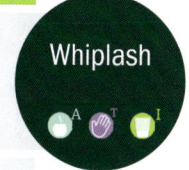

Withdrawal Symptoms
[A T I]

- Daily Tea [I]
- Detoxification Blend [A T I]
- Grapefruit [A T I]
- Cinnamon [A T I]
- Juniper Berry [A T I]

Apply 1-3 drops to bottoms of feet and back of neck; inhale from cupped hands as needed; add 1-3 drops to water.

Workout Enhancement
[A T I]

Protocol on pg. 163

Use caps, powders, and protein to enhance workouts for building muscle and losing weight.

- Advanced Thermogenic Caps [I]
- AM Exercise Caps [I]
- Limitless Energy Powder [I]
- Moringa Plant Protein [I]
- Pre-Workout Powder [I]

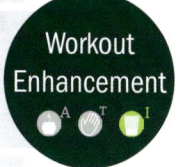

Worms
[A T I]

- Oregano [T I]
- Patchouli [T I]
- Immunity-Boosting Blend [T I]
- Thyme [T I]
- Clove [T I]

Apply 2-4 drops to stomach area and on bottoms of feet 2 or 3 times daily; ingest 2-3 drops twice daily.

Wrinkles
[A T I]

Use Moringa-enhanced skin products. Apply 1-3 drops of oil to the affected areas as needed. Add to facial lotion or use with carrier oil for added benefits.

- Moringa Skin Products [T]
- Skin-Enriching Blend [T]
- Myrrh [T]
- Frankincense [T]
- Sandalwood [T]

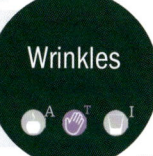

Ailments

○ Aromatic   ○ Topical   ○ Internal

45

Nutritionals

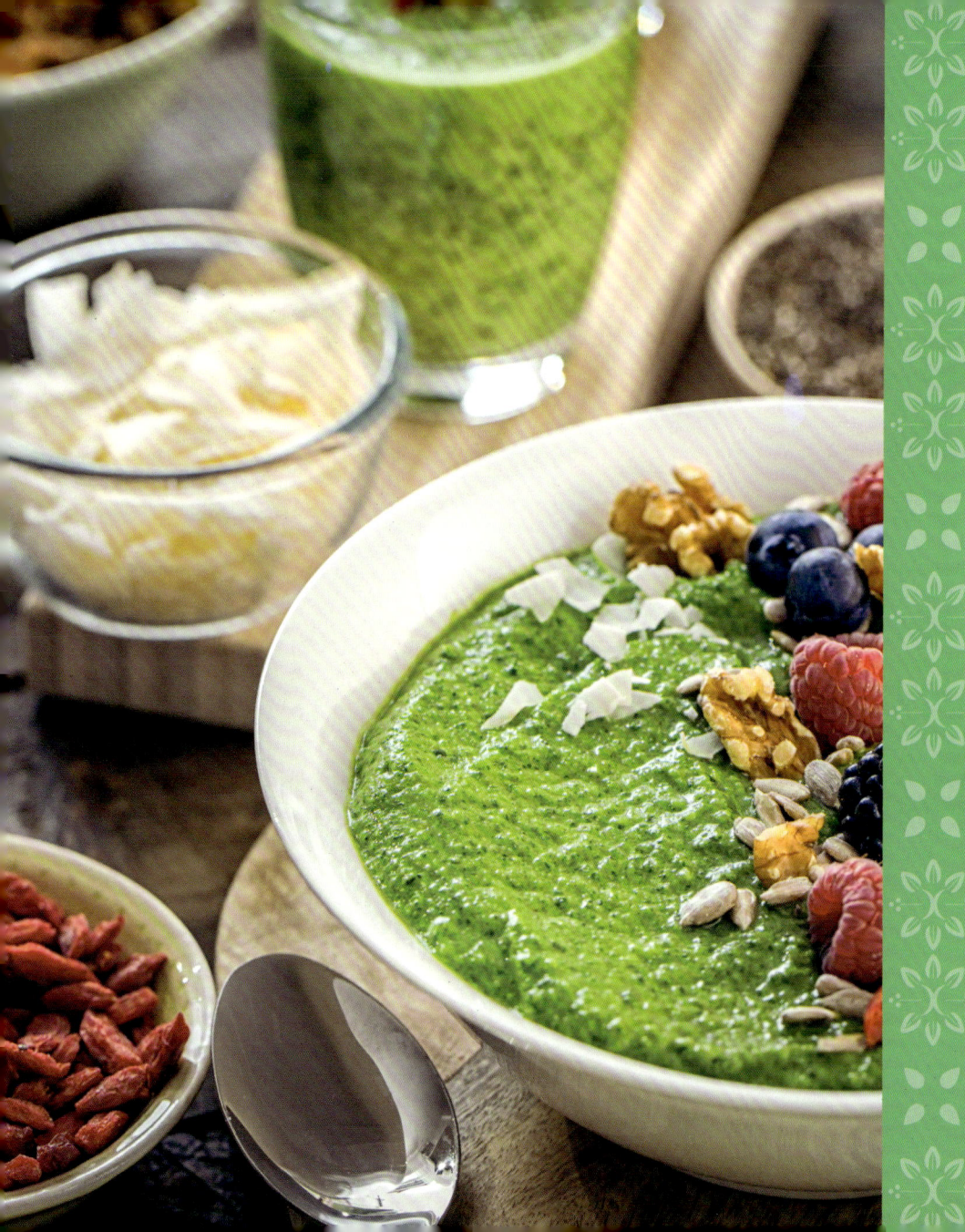

Advanced Thermogenic Caps

known name

Key Ingredients
Niacinamide (B3), Methylcobalamin (B12), Calcium, Phosphorus, Natural Caffeine, N-Acetyl Cysteine, Green Tea Extract, Moringine HCl, Hordenine HCl, Trimethylglycine, Advantra Z

Key Uses
- Boosts basal metabolic rate
- Increases efficacy of strenuous exercise
- Targets weight loss
- Harnesses Energy
- Controls appetite

Why it Works

Using thermogenic supplements increases your body's natural ability to harness energy. You might feel heat or a slight tingling as the supplement begins to activate.

Using a thermogenic supplement with strenuous exercise helps train your body to permanently maintain a higher metabolism.

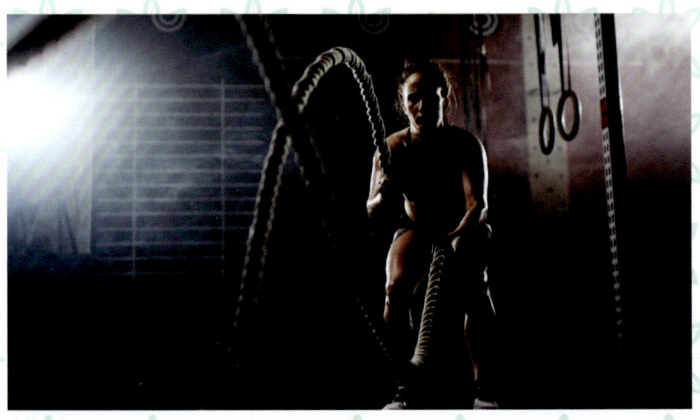

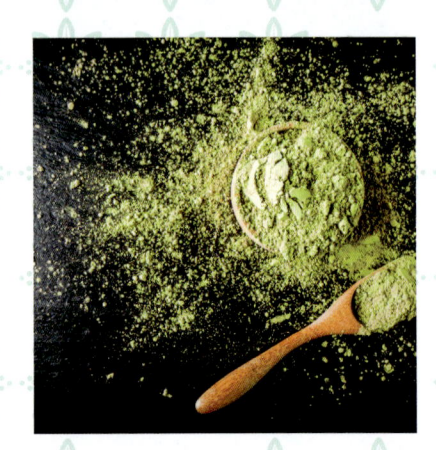

Nutritionals

48

AM Exercise Enhancing Caps

known name

Key Ingredients
Green Coffee Bean, Natural Caffeine, Rhodiola Rosea, Citrus Aurantium, Moringa Oleifera Blend

Key Uses
- Curbs appetite and encourages smarter food choices
- Provides the body with 90+ key nutrients
- Boosts energy and mood naturally

Why it Works

Providing the body with fuel and natural energy-enhancing agents increases the desire to be active. Supplementing to improve mood does the same.

This exercise-enhancing supplement not only improves the feeling of exercise, it helps get you out the door to begin with.

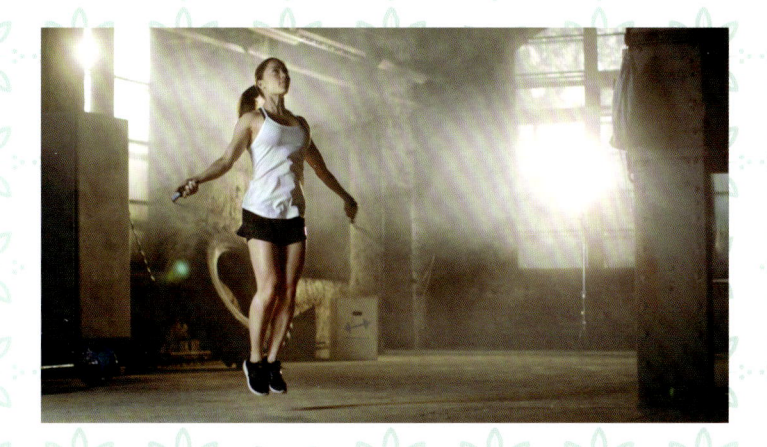

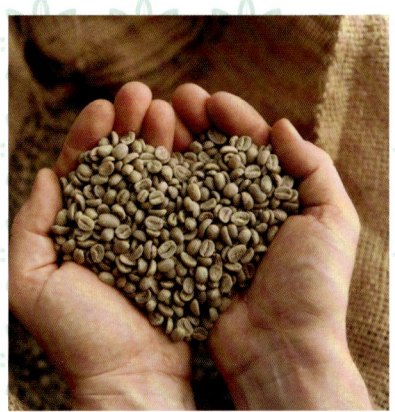

Nutritionals

Daily Tea

known name

Key Ingredients
Garninia Cambogia Extract, Bitter Melon Extract, Ginger Root, Orange Peel, Astragalus Root, Bilberry Leaf, Stevia, Moringa Oleifera Blend

Key Uses
- Promotes feelings of fullness
- Keeps in line with true caloric needs
- Triggers serotonin release to promote feelings of satiation
- Blocks fat absorption
- De-stresses cells

Why it Works

Hunger is an indicator of a physical need, while cravings are a desire for mental stimulation. This herbal tea helps maintain a sense of satisfaction, collectedness, and calm.

As you feel satisfied, you're more likely to eat according to your true caloric needs.

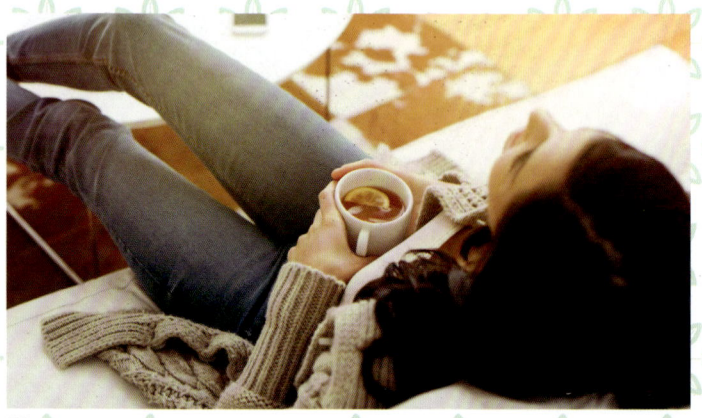

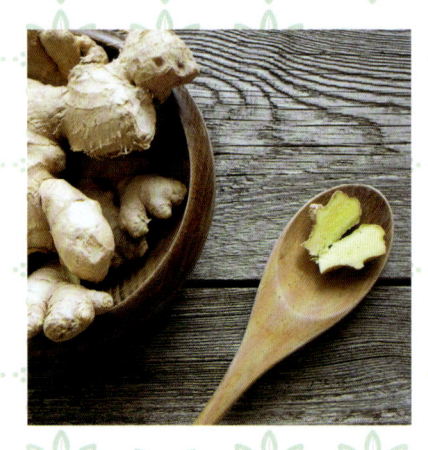

Nutritionals

During Workout Fuel

known name

Key Ingredients
Glucose, Fructose, L-Arginine, Citric Acid, Silica, Ribose, Sodium Chloride, Stearic Acid, Malic Acid, Dipotassium Phosphate, Stevia, Beet Root, Elderberry

Key Uses
- Increases blood flow
- Provides quick-absorbing energy to cells and muscles
- Replenishes electrolytes

Why it Works

Replenishing electrolytes allows the body to maintain better communication between cells and systems, maintain osmotic regulation, and it facilitates key enzymatic reactions.

Muscles and organs respond quickly to the mono-saccharides and electrolytes found in this supplement.

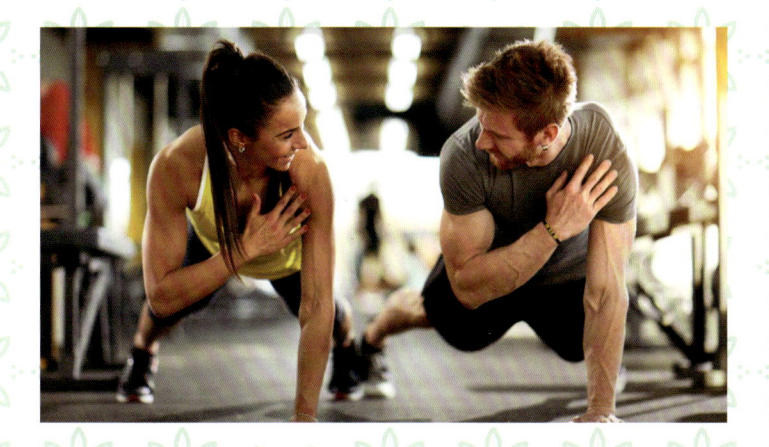

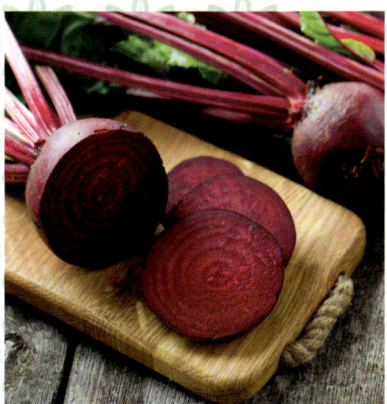

Nutritionals

Energy Drink Supplement

known name

Key Ingredients
Purified Water, Moringa Oleifera Blend, Sugar, Citric Acid, Malic Acid, Natural Caffeine, Sodium Chloride, Silica, Stevia, DiPotassium Phosphate, Elderberry, Brigham Tea, Green Tea, Ginseng, Garlic

Key Uses
- Boosts mood
- Increases endurance
- Suppresses appetite
- Easily accessible, portable energy

Why it Works

This ready-to-consume beverage activates the body differently from store-bought stimulants. Its stimulating agents are accompanied by a complex array of plant-derived nutrients.

Providing the body with a complex and more complete source of fuel allows it to perform without the unhealthy jitters from ordinary caffeine stimulants.

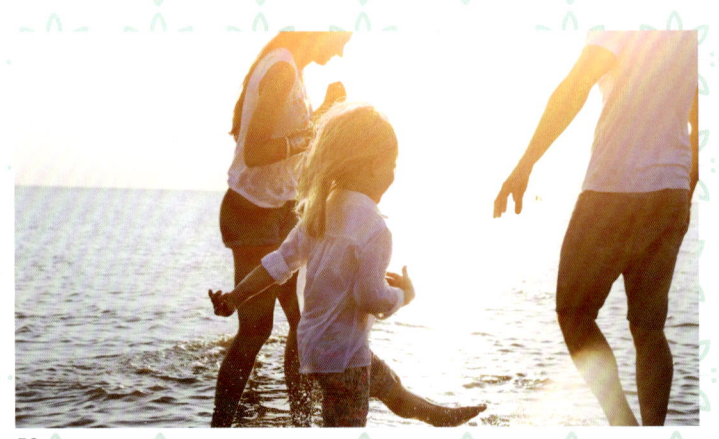

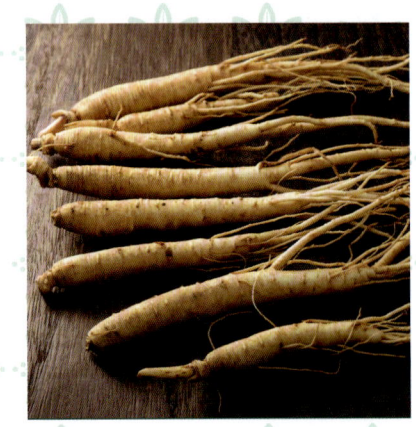

Extreme Moringa Capsules

known name

Key Ingredients
Green Tea, DMHA, Natural Caffeine, KinetiQ, Caffeine Citrate, Korean Ginseng, Niacin, Hordinine, Moringine, Evodiamine, Trimethylglycine, FloGard, Rice Flour, BioPerene® , Gelatin Capsule

Key Uses
- Improves focus
- Increases energy
- Suppresses appetite
- Provides the benefits of Moringa with the benefits of other accompanying herbs

Why it Works

This supplement provides the stimulating and energizing benefits of extracts from the Moringa plant and other trusted herbs.

The combination of caffeine with other plant-based stimulants provides a stable source of focus and energy. It also provides a boost for recovery functions in the body.

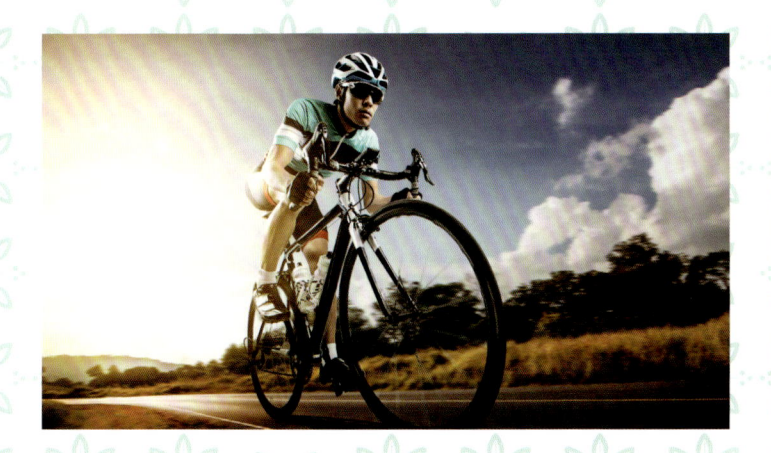

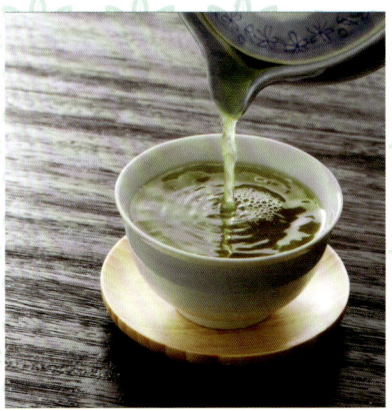

Nutritionals

Extreme Moringa Energy

known name

Key Ingredients
Moringa Leaf, Natural Flavor, Ephedra Nevadensis, Green Tea Extract, Moringa Seed, Moringa Fruit, Ginseng, Garlic, Cane Sugar, Fruit Pectin, Citric Acid, Mango Flavoring, Natural Caffeine, Agar, Stevia, Silica, Stearic Acid

Key Uses
- Increases metabolic energy
- Aids in weight loss
- Helps control appetite
- Supports healthy cellular function
- Increases cardiovascular capacity
- Improves oxygenation and circulation
- Provides fast-acting and long-lasting energy

Why it Works

Obtaining energy from food is always a more sustainable practice than using market-popular stimulants.

This energy supplement uses scientifically balanced combinations of plant-derived nutrients to provide reliable energy without the crash of harmful neurostimulants.

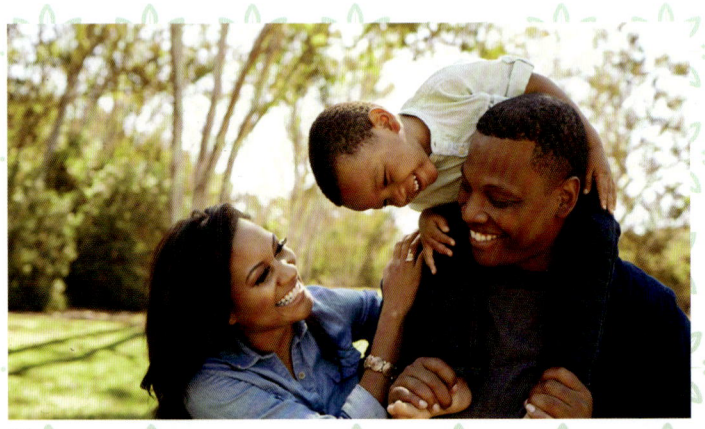

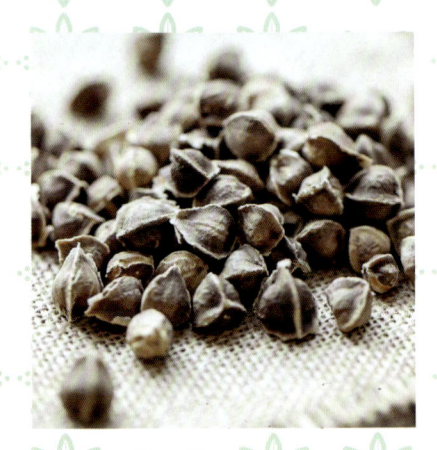

Nutritionals

Hydration Powder

known name

Key Ingredients
Glucose, Fructose, Natural Flavor, Citric Acid, Malic Acid, Sodium Chloride, Silica, Stevia, Dipotassium Phosphate, Stearic Acid, Beet Juice Powder, Elderberry Powder

Key Uses
- Replaces soda and sugary sport drinks
- Contains 1/10th the calories of a large soda
- Replenishes electrolytes
- Colored from beet juice powder and elderberries

Why it Works
This soda and sports drink alternative provides the satisfaction of a flavored drink without harmful amounts of sugar. It's safe for adults and children of all ages.

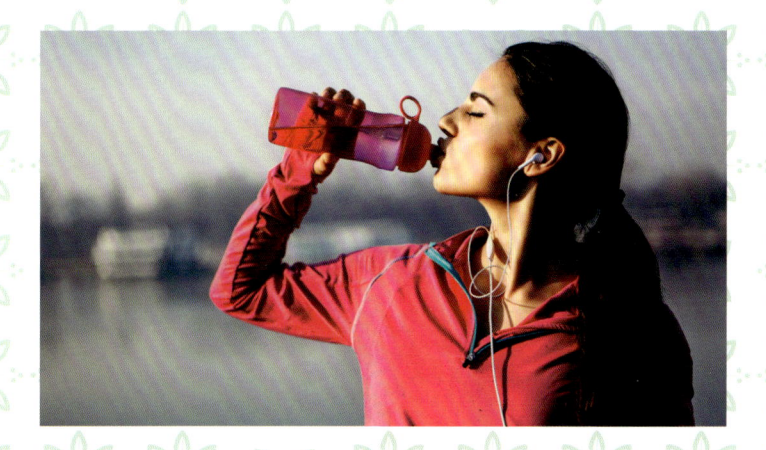

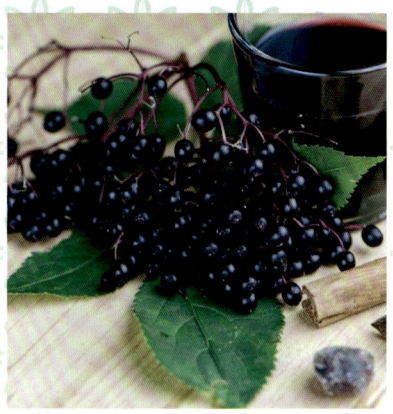

Nutritionals

Limitless Energy Powder

known name

Key Ingredients
Coconut Juice Powder, L-Arginine, gamma-Aminobutyric Acid (GABA), D-Ribose, Natural Caffeine, Carrot Root Powder, Taurine, Apple Extract, Korean Ginseng Root Extract, Moringa oleifera Blend (Leaf Powder, Seed Cake, Fruit Powder), Mangosteen Fruit Powder, Beet Root Powder, Elderberry Juice Powder, Garlic Powder, Ginger Root Extract, Gotu Kola 4:1 Extract

Key Uses
- Easy on-the-go energy boost
- Replenishes electrolytes
- Increases alertness & mental clarity
- Supports peak muscle performance
- Supports nerve responses
- Improves mood

Why it Works

This blend combines Moringa, Mangosteen, D-Ribose, and GABA for a boost that feels amazing.

It's like jump starting your muscles and mind while simultaneously providing the zen of fluid and mood balance.

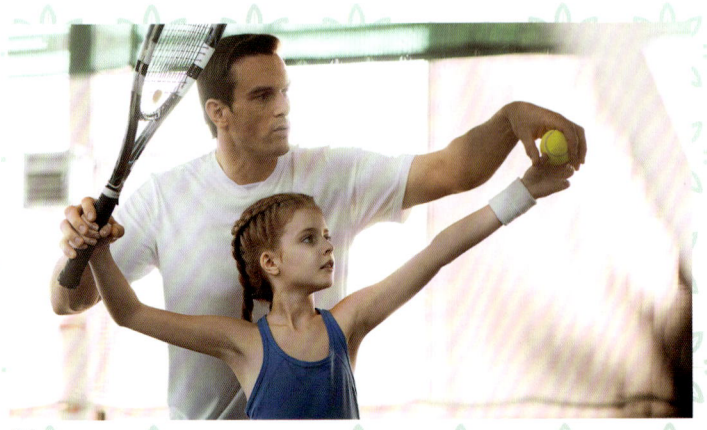

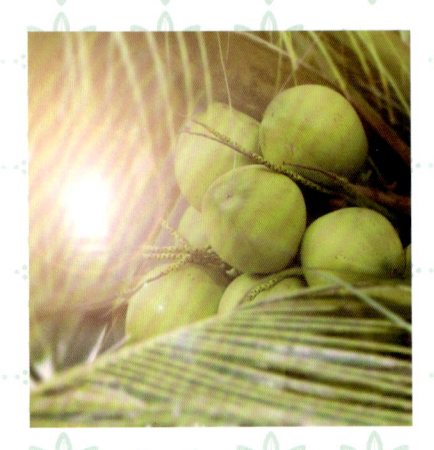

Moringa Super Powder

known name

Key Ingredients
Moringa Proprietary Blend (Moringa Oleifera Leaf Powder, Seed Cake, & Fruit Powder), Cane Sugar, Fruit Pectin, Agar, Citric Acid, Stevia, Silica

Key Uses
- 90+ verifiable cell-ready crucial nutrients, antioxidants, minerals, omega oils, & proteins
- Provides natural energy
- Increases focus
- Supports healthy inflammatory response
- Helps curb appetite
- Ideal for weight loss
- Nourishes the immune system
- Helps maintain healthy blood sugar levels
- Promotes healthy circulation
- Supports healthy digestion
- Provides natural anti-aging benefits

Why it Works

Healthy bodies get their nutrition from plants, and the healthiest get it from superplants.

Moringa Oleifera combats nutritional famine by providing one of the most complex and balanced blends of nutrients found in nature. Use it daily as the core of ideal, plant-based nutrition.

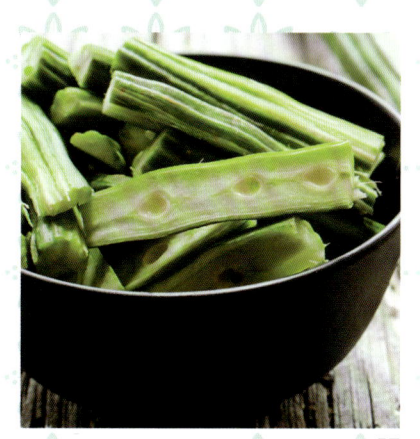

Nutritionals

Moringa + Whey Protein Powder

known name

Key Ingredients
Whey Protein, Moringa Oleifera Blend, Flavoring, Cane Sugar, Stevia, Fruit Pectin

Key Uses
- Provides protein and fiber to build lean muscle
- Rebuilds muscle fibers
- Boosts energy with nutrients provided by moringa

Why it Works

Certain nutrients needed for energy production and building muscle mass operate more effectively when accompanied by other complimenting nutrients.

This protein blend provides industry-standard whey protein with a blend of nutrients that make the protein more usable in the body.

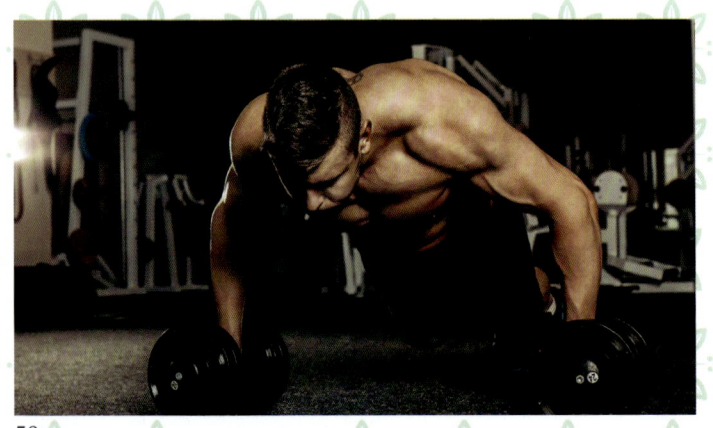

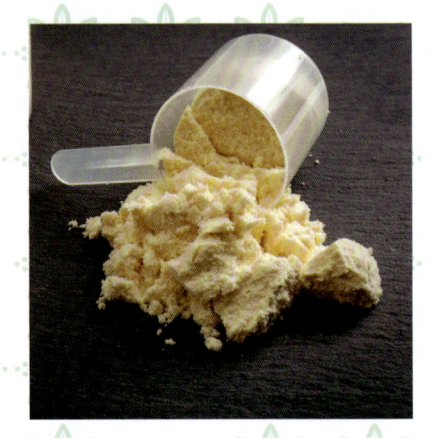

Nitric Oxide Activator

known name

Key Ingredients
Moringa Blend, Beet Root Extract, Hawthorn Berry, L-Citrulline, Green Tea Powder, Red Spinach Extract, Beet Root Powder, Pomegranate Fruit Extract, Shishsandra Chinensis Berry Extract, Celery Seed Extract

Key Uses
- Delivers oxygen to muscles, tissues, and organs
- Supports cardiovascular performance
- Increases cardiovascular longevity
- Increases circulation
- Ideal for cold extremities
- Vasodilator properties can help with impotence
- Improves mental activity & memory
- Helps regulate blood pressure

Why it Works
Nitric Oxide Activator allows oxygen and crucial nutrients to be effectively delivered throughout the body. It facilitates optimal function of body system relations, allowing body systems to work more synergistically together.

Using this activator daily feels like speeding up the productivity at the factory.

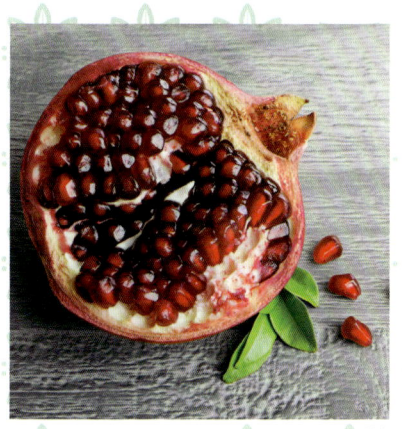

Nutritionals

Optimal Aging Formula

known name

Key Ingredients
Moringa Blend, Baikal Skullcap Root, White Korean Ginseng, Immortality Herb Root

Key Uses
- Promotes optimal aging
- Combats premature signs of aging
- Provides anti-inflammatory support
- Harnesses traditional Asian medicine for life longevity
- Increases energy, endurance, stamina, and recovery

Why it Works
This blend reduces unhealthy inflammation at a cellular level. Reducing inflammation allows cells, organs, and body systems to operate and regenerate optimally. This allows the body to feel and function better while increasing lifetime longevity.

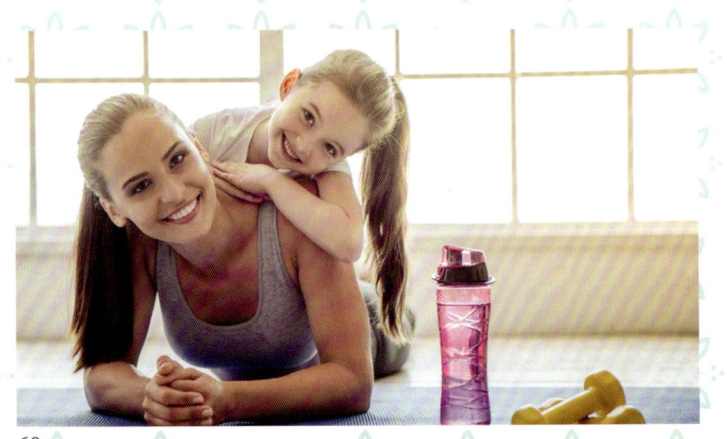

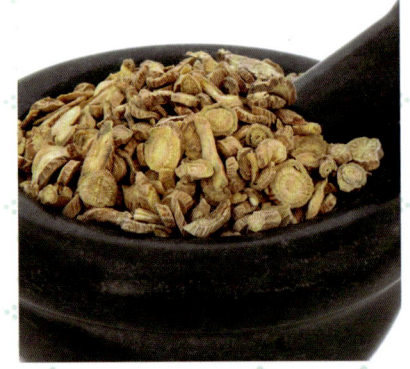

Plant Protein

known name

Key Ingredients
Pea Protein, Rice Protein, Moringa Leaf Protein, Xylotol, Natural Flavors, sunflower Lecithin, Medium Chain Triglycerides, Stevia, Sodium Chloride

Key Uses
- Provides a complete protein exclusively from plant sources
- Meets needs for all nine essential amino acids
- Gluten-free, soy-free, and vegan

Why it Works

This protein provides a complete array of the essential amino acids needed for building lean muscle and maintaining healthy energy levels.

Unlike many plant proteins that utilize only pea or rice, this is a complex and highly bio-available plant protein that can be used on an ongoing basis.

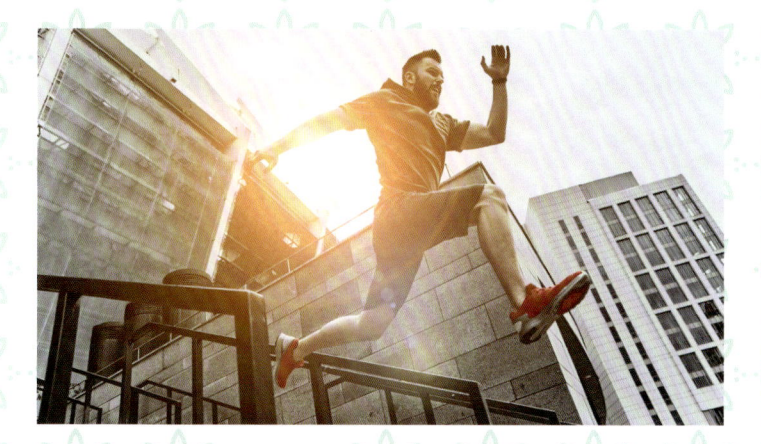

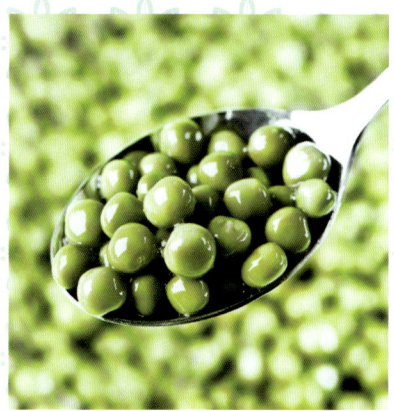

Nutritionals

PM Craving Control Caps

known name

Key Ingredients
Gymnema Sylvestre Extract, Trim Blend, Ashwagandha Root Extract, Atlantic Kelp, Moringa Oleifera Blend, 5-HTP, Vanaduim, Silica, Magnesium Stearate, Chromium

Key Uses
- Aids digestion and weight loss
- Promotes a calm mind and body
- Decreases sugar cravings

Why it Works

The extracts in this blend help control evening cravings while preparing the body for more restful sleep.

Using it consistently helps train the body when to expect food and when to expect meaningful rest.

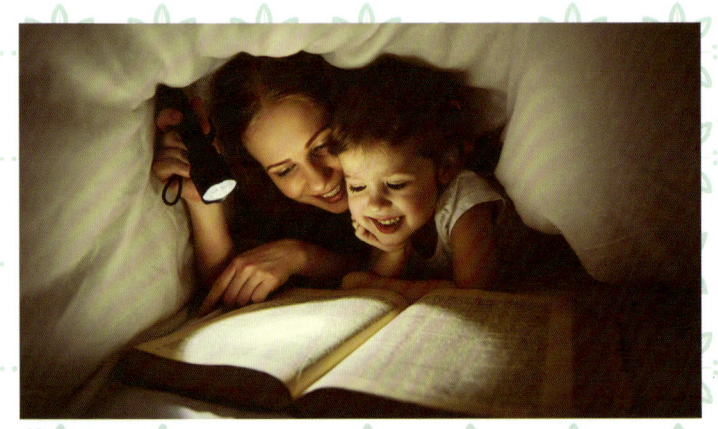

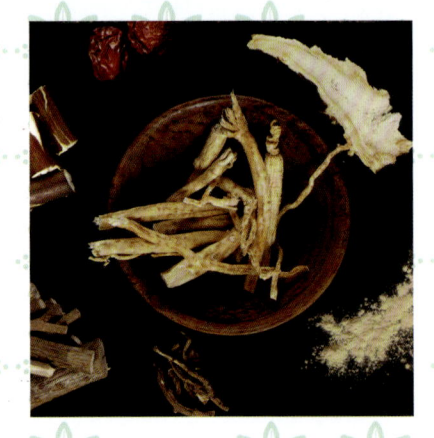

Nutritionals

Post-Workout Powder

known name

Key Ingredients
Garninia Cambogia Extract, Bitter Melon Extract, Ginger Root, Orange Peel, Astragalus Root, Bilberry Leaf, Stevia, Moringa Oleifera Blend

Key Uses
- Removes lactic acid from muscles to prevent reactive oxygen species
- Provides branch chain amino acids (BCAAs)
- Provides lubrication and protection to joints & cartilage
- Provides antioxidants

Why it Works

This powder provides Branch Chain Amino Acids (BCAAs in ideal ratios, helping muscles to respond positively to aggressive exercise. It also helps flush out lactic acid after working out. The result is quicker recovery and more effective muscle building.

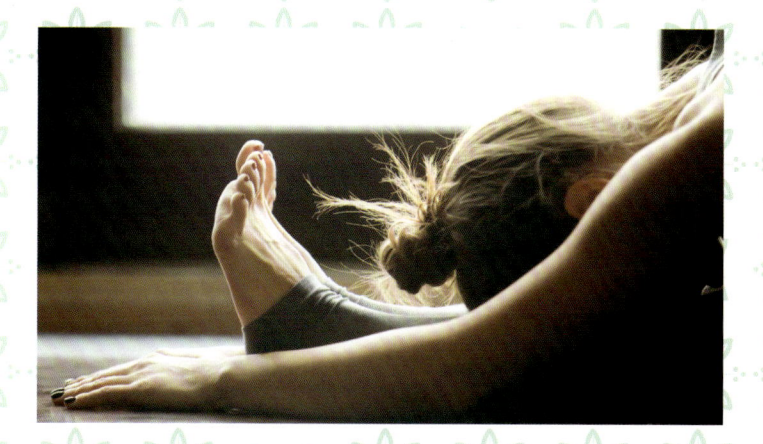

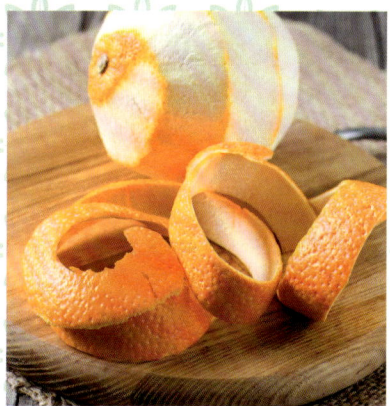

Nutritionals

Pre-Workout Powder

known name

Key Ingredients
Natural Flavor, Beta-Alanine, L-Arginine, Citric Acid, L-Carnitine, Potassium Bicarbonate, Stevia, Natural Caffeine, Synephrine HCl, Yohimbine, Creatine, Elderberry, Niacin, Rhodiola Rosea, B12

Key Uses
- Optimizes metabolic performance
- Get more out of workouts
- Initiates blood flow
- Heightens thermogenic response

Why it Works

The safe, natural stimulants in this pre-workout effectively prepare the body for activity. It's designed to promote physiological and metabolic optimization, making exercise more likely and more productive.

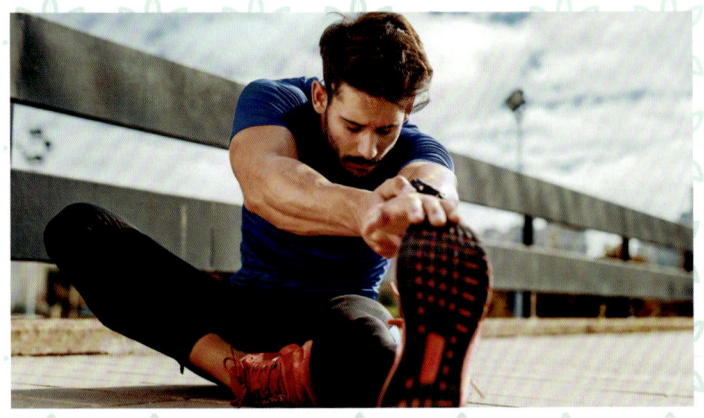

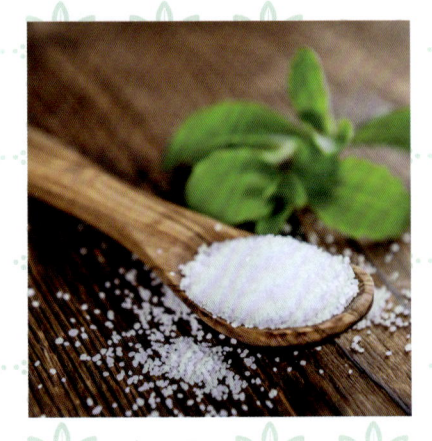

Nutritionals

Premium Tea

known name

Key Ingredients
Senna Leaf, Buckthorn Frang Bark, Peppermint Leaf, Stevia Leaf, Uva Ursi Leaf, Orange Peel, Rose Hips Fruit, Althea Root, Moringa Oleifera Blend, Chamomile Flower

Key Uses
- Eliminates toxins from fat cells
- Supports digestive health
- Detoxes organs and cells
- Promotes feeling fuller longer

Why it Works

This tea uses gentle, safe, natural herbs to help the body flush out toxins and harmful agents that get built up from dietary and environmental conditions.

Frequent detoxification allows the body to utilize fat stores as energy, absorb nutrients from food, and direct nutrients and energy to healthy systemic functions.

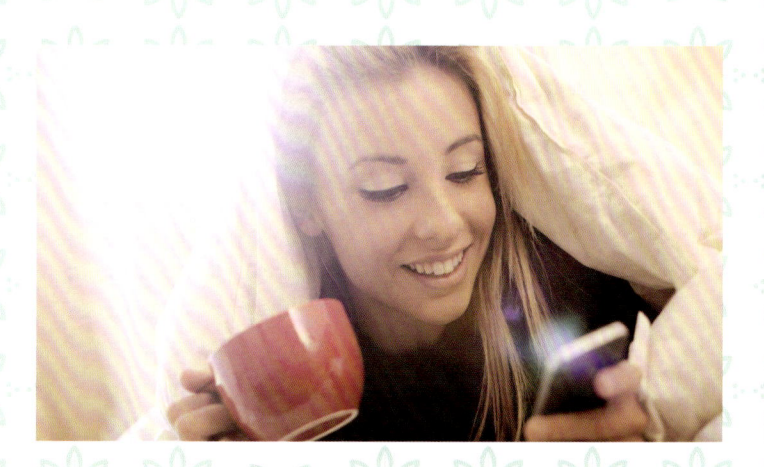

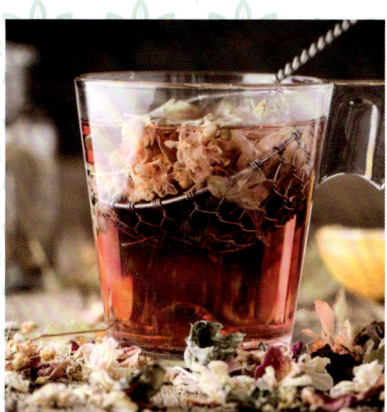

Nutritionals

Single Oils

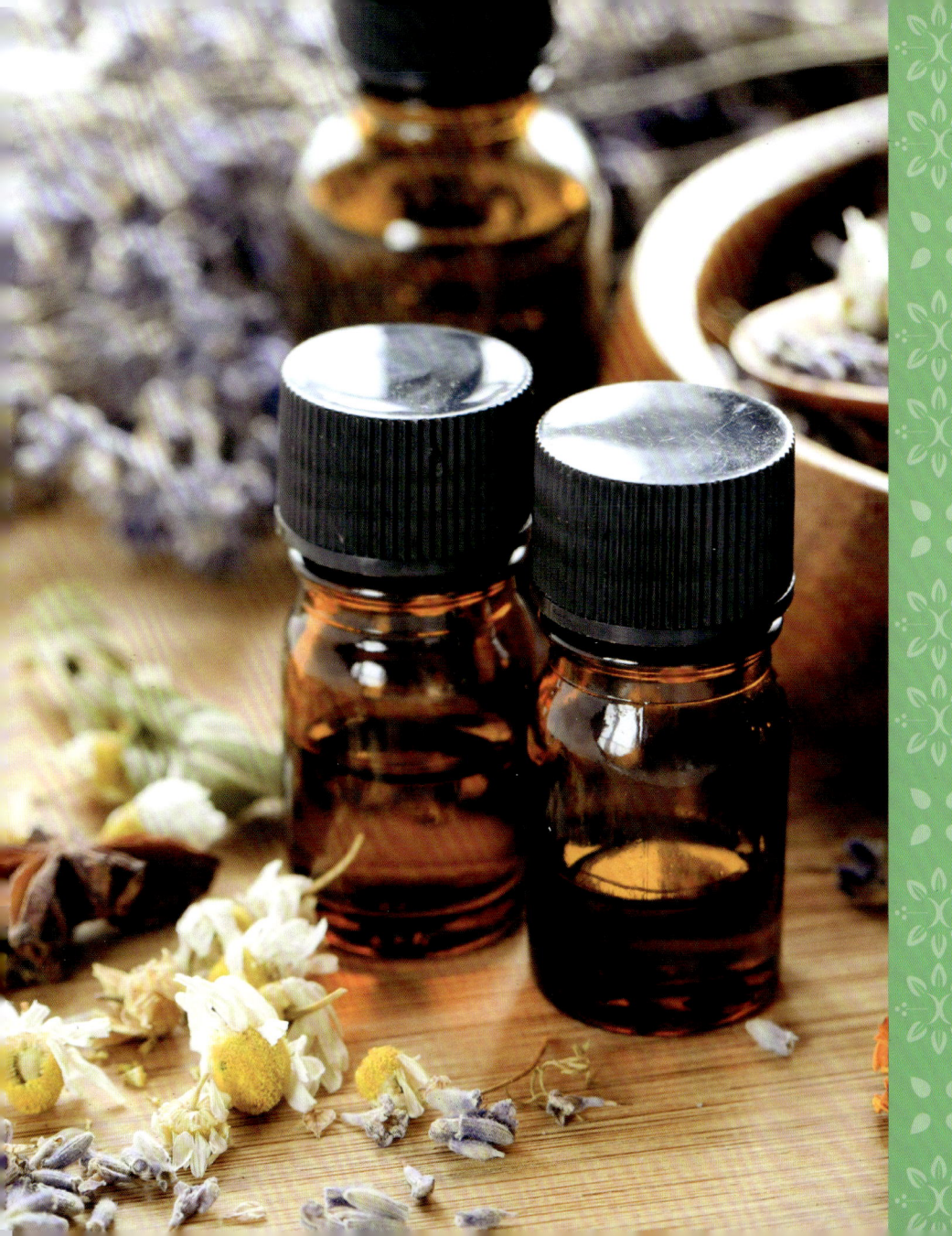

Atlas Cedarwood
Cedrus Atlantica

Top Uses

ADD/ADHD
Apply 1-3 drops to wrists, temples, and back of neck, or diffuse.

Eczema & Psoriasis
Apply neat and often to affected areas.

Sleep
Rub onto bottoms of feet, the back of neck, and over top of pillow. Blend with lavender for added effect.

Anxiety
Apply to wrists and temples, or inhale from cupped hands.

Seizures & Strokes
Apply 1-3 drops to back of neck and bottoms of feet.

Cuts & Scrapes
Apply around wounded area to promote tissue healing.

Application

Safety
Safe for neat application.

Key Properties
Antiseptic
Anti-inflammatory
Diuretic
Astringent
Insecticidal

Other Uses
Bladder Infection, Blemishes, Cough, Dandruff, Gums, Insect Repellent, Respiratory Health, Sinusitis, Tension, Urinary Infection, Vaginal Infection

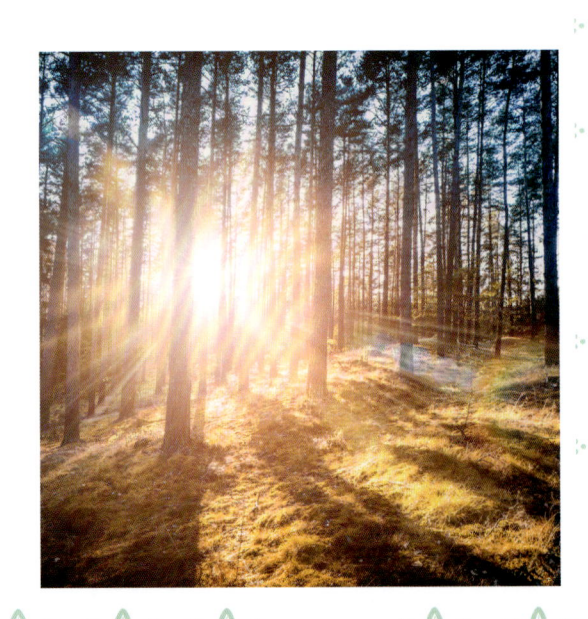

Balsam Fir
Abies Balsamea

Top Uses

Muscle Soreness
Rub 2-4 drops with carrier oil onto sore muscles.

Headache & Migraine
Rub a drop into temples.

Congestion
Rub 1-2 drops over chest, or diffuse.

Focus & Mental Clarity
Inhale from cupped hands, or diffuse several drops.

Skin Irritations
Apply heavily diluted to skin irritations and rashes.

Household Cleaning
Use with Lemon oil for a refreshing and natural household cleaner.

Constipation
Take 1-3 drops in water or a capsule, or rub onto outside of stomach.

Application

Safety
Safe for neat application.

Key Properties
Analgesic
Antioxidant
Anti-catarrhal
Tonic
Antimicrobial

Other Uses
Arthritis, Depression, Emotional Congestion, Energy, Generational Healing, Weight Gain, Sinus Issues

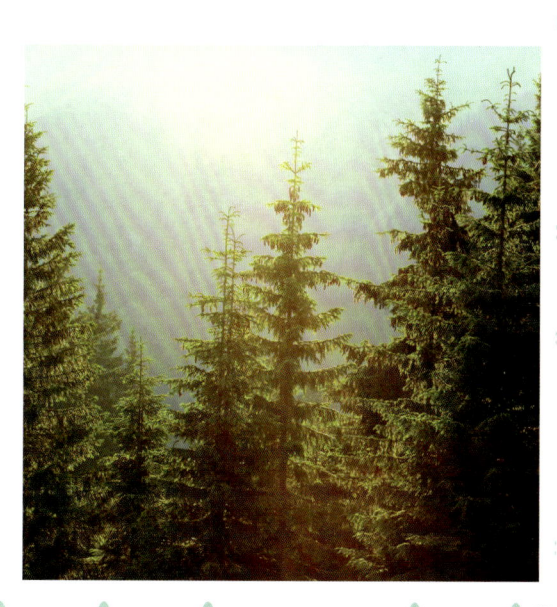

Single Oils

69

Basil (sweet)
Ocimum Basilicum

Top Uses

Mental Fatigue
Inhale from cupped hands, or diffuse several drops.

Adrenal Fatigue
Massage 1-2 drops directly over adrenal areas, or onto the bottoms of feet.

Carpal Tunnel
Massage 1-2 drops into wrists & joints.

Earache
Place a drop on a cotton ball, and rest over the ear for 15 minutes.

Muscle Spasms
Massage 2-4 drops diluted into muscles.

Cramps (abdominal)
Rub a drop clockwise over abdomen.

Cooking
Add a toothpick swirl to achieve desired flavor.

Application

Key Properties
Neurotonic
Regenerative
Antispasmodic
Neurotonic
Steroidal

Other Uses
Bee Stings, Bronchitis, Dizziness, Frozen Shoulder, Gout, Greasy Hair, Infertility, Lactation (increase milk supply), Loss of Sense of Smell, Migraines, Nausea, Viral Hepatitis

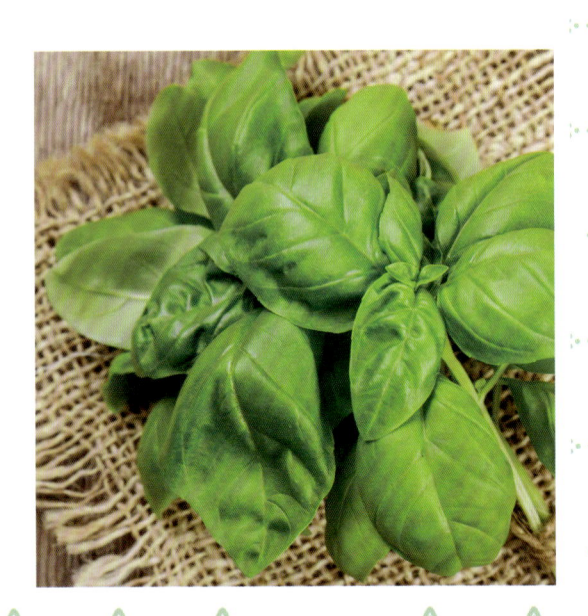

Safety
Dilute for sensitive skin. Use with caution if pregnant or epileptic.

Bergamot
Citrus Bergamia

Top Uses

Sadness & Depression
Inhale a few drops from cupped hands, or diffuse.

Psoriasis
Dilute 1-2 drops heavily in carrier oil, and apply often to affected area.

Addictions
Apply 2-4 drops to bottoms of feet, or diffuse.

Appetite Loss
Drink 1-3 drops in water throughout the day. Also diffuse.

Self Confidence/Self-Worth
Apply over sacral area (middle section).

Insomnia
Use a drop under tongue or in water 30 minutes before bed.

Application

Safety
Avoid UV exposure 12 hours after topical use.

Key Properties
Antidepressant
Anti-inflammatory
Neurotonic
Antibacterial
Digestive

Other Uses
Acne, Brain Injury, Colic, Depression, Fungal Infections, Irritability, Low Energy, Muscle Cramps, Oily Skin, Stress

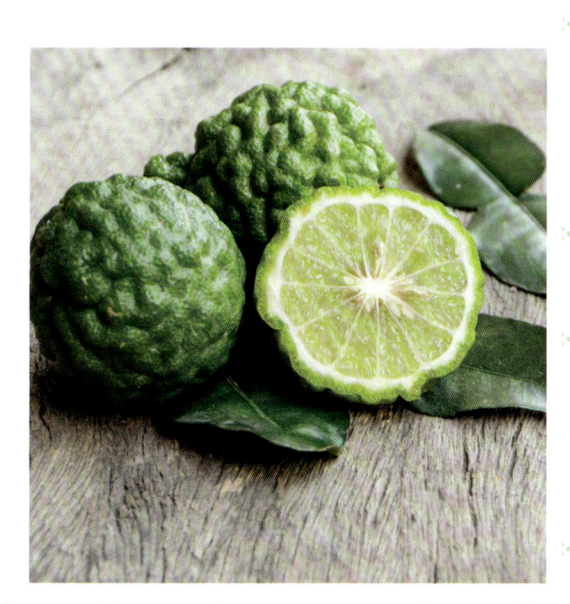

Black Pepper
Piper Nigrum

Application

Safety
Dilute for use on sensitive skin.

Top Uses

Muscle Spasms & Sprains
Massage 2-4 drops into muscles with carrier oil.

Cold & Flu
Take 2-4 drops in a capsule, or apply to the bottoms of feet.

Circulation
Apply 2-4 drops to bottoms of feet.

Smoking Addiction
Apply 1-3 drops to bottoms of feet (big toes) several times a day to curb cravings.

Congestion
Apply 1-3 drops diluted over chest and upper back.

Airborne Viruses
Diffuse several drops to cleanse the air.

Cooking
Add a drop to soups, sauces, and other dishes.

Key Properties
Antioxidant
Antispasmodic
Expectorant
Nerurotonic
Rubefacient

Other Uses
Antioxidant, Anxiety, Cellular Oxygenation, Diarrhea, Digestion, Gas, Emotional Addiction, Emotional Repression, Inflammation, Laxative

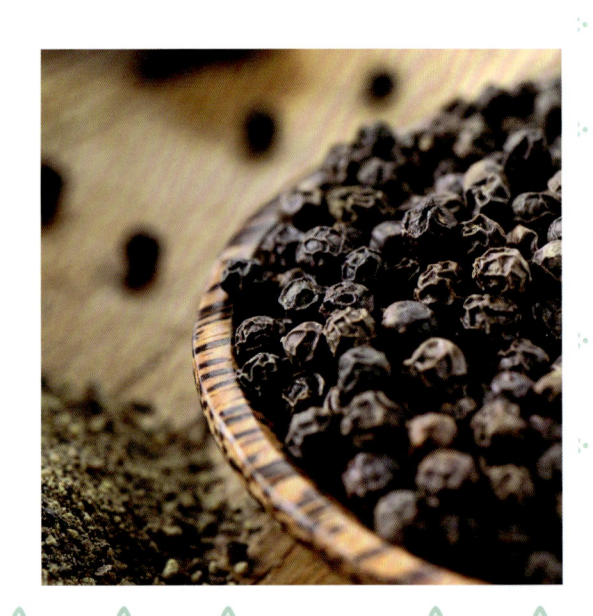

Blue Tansy
Tanacetum Annuum

Top Uses

Anxiety
Apply a drop to pulse points, or diffuse.

Allergies
Apply 1-3 drops to bottoms of feet, inhale from cupped hands, or diffuse.

Arthritis & Muscle Pain
Add 5-10 drops to a bath, or massage into affected areas with carrier oil.

Digestive Discomfort
Rub a drop with carrier oil clockwise onto stomach.

Dry, Itchy, or Inflamed Skin
Apply heavily diluted to affected areas.

Congestion
Rub a drop diluted onto chest and mid-back.

Headaches
Massage a drop diluted onto temples and base of skull.

Application

Safety
Dilute heavily to avoid temporary blue staining.

Key Properties
Anti-histamine
Anti-allergenic
Anti-fungal
Vermicide
Stomachic

Other Uses
Bacterial Infections, Constipation, Cramping, Eczema, Fungus, Gas, Gout, Indigestion, Insect Repellent, Psoriasis, Rashes, Rheumatism, Sneezing

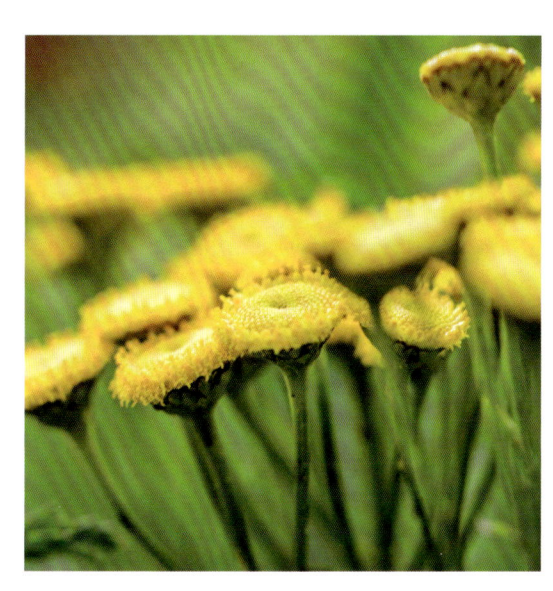

Cinnamon
Cinnamomum Verum

Top Uses

Diabetes
Take 1-2 drops in a capsule daily.

Sex Drive
Use heavily diluted in massage, or diffuse several drops.

Bacterial Infections
Apply heavily diluted for external infection, or take 1-2 drops in a capsule a few times a day for internal infection.

Cavities
Swish a drop with water as a mouthwash.

Alkalinity
Drink a drop in water to promote alkalinity.

High Blood Sugar
Take 1-2 drops in a capsule, or drink with a large glass of water.

Application

Safety
Dilute for topical use. Avoid during pregnancy.

Key Properties
Antiviral
Antimicrobial
Antiseptic
Antioxidant
Aphrodisiac

Other Uses
Airborne Bacteria, Cholesterol, Diverticulitis, Fungal Infections, General Tonic, Immune Support, Pancreas Support, Pneumonia, Typhoid, Vaginitis

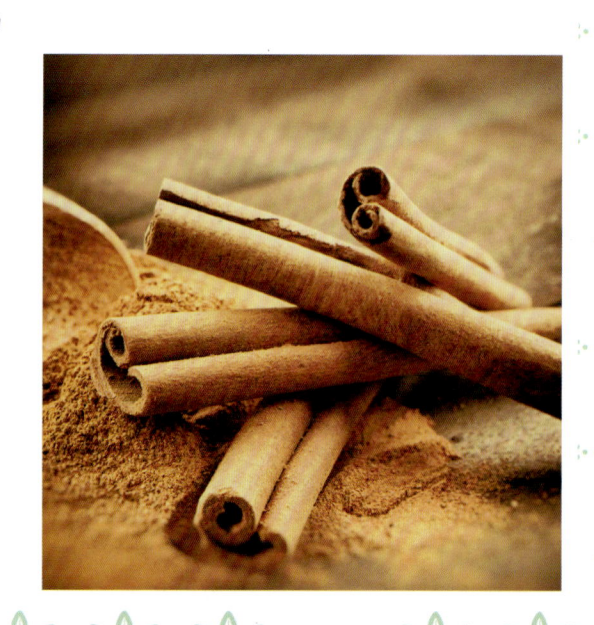

Clary Sage
Salvia Sclarea

Top Uses

PMS
Apply to bottoms of feet, or take 1-2 drops in a capsule.

Hormone Balance
Apply 1-2 drops to wrists and behind ears.

Postpartum Depression
Diffuse or apply over heart area.

Abdominal Cramps
Massage 1-3 drops over abdomen.

Infertility
Apply to abdomen & uterine reflex points, or take 1-2 drops in a capsule.

Breast Cancer
Apply diluted to breasts a few times a day, and take 1-2 drops in a capsule to regulate estrogen levels.

Pink Eye
Apply a dab carefully around edge of eye.

Application

Safety
Use with caution during pregnancy.

Key Properties
Emmenagogue
Galactagogue
Mucolytic
Sedative
Antispasmodic

Other Uses
Aneurysm, Breast Enlargement, Cholesterol, Convulsions, Endometriosis, Epilepsy, Fragile Hair, Hot Flashes, Impotence, Lactation, Parkinson's, Premenopause, Seizure

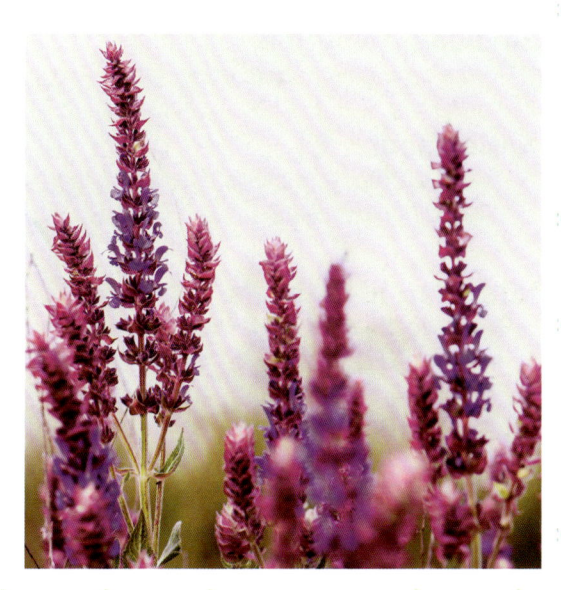

Clove
Syzgium Aromaticum

Top Uses

Toothache
Apply a drop directly to affected tooth.

Thyroid (hypo, Hashimoto's)
Apply 1-2 drops diluted over thyroid or to thyroid reflex point, or take in capsule.

Immune Support
Take 1-2 drops in a capsule.

Smoking Addiction
Rub a drop onto bottom of big toe.

Antioxidant
Take 1-2 drops in a capsule, or use a toothpick swirl in cooking.

Rheumatoid Arthritis
Massage 1-2 drops diluted into affected area.

Liver Detox
Rub 1-3 drops diluted over liver or on liver reflex point.

Application

Safety
Use with caution during pregnancy. Dilute for sensitive skin.

Key Properties
Antioxidant
Antiviral
Nervine
Antibacterial
Anti-parasitic

Other Uses
Addictions, Blood Clots, Candida, Cataracts, Fever, Herpes Simplex, Hodgkin's Disease, Glaucoma, Gingivitis, Lipoma, Lupus, Lyme Disease, Macular Degeneration, Memory Loss, Parasites, Termites

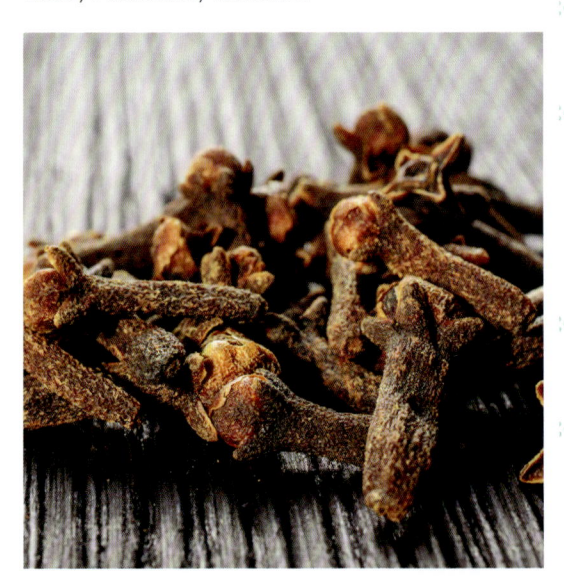

Copaiba
Copaifera Officinalis

Top Uses

Pain & Inflammation
Use 1-2 drops under the tongue, or apply topically to affected areas.

Headache & Migraine
Massage gently onto temples, scalp, and back of neck.

Wrinkles, Blisters, & Pimples
Apply a drop to affected areas a few times a day.

Detox
Apply 2-4 drops over bladder to stimulate detox through urination.

High Blood Pressure
Apply to the bottoms of feet twice daily.

Athlete's Foot
Apply several drops to clean, dry feet.

Cancer & Autoimmune Disorders
Take 2-4 drops in a capsule 3-4 times a day, and apply along spine at night.

Application

Safety
Safe for neat application.

Key Properties
Analgesic
Anti-inflammatory
Anti-carcinoma
Carminative
Anti-arthritic

Other Uses
Anxiety, Blisters, Congestion, Endometriosis, Gout, Infection, Intestinal Infections, Liver Toxicity, Mood Disorders, Nail Fungus, Scar Tissue, Sleep Issues, Skin Strengthening, Tendinitis, Tonsillitis

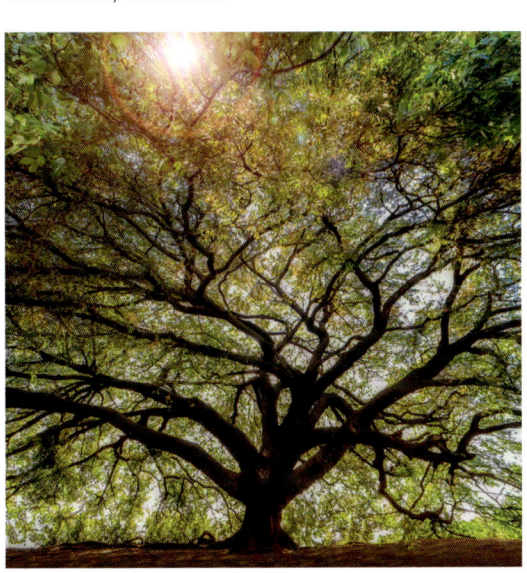

Coriander
Coriandrum Sativum

Application

Safety
Safe for neat application.

Top Uses

Cartilage Injury
Massage 1-3 drops into affected area with carrier oil.

Diabetes (high blood sugar)
Combine 1 drop with 1 drop Cinnamon & Juniper Berry in a capsule daily.

Body Odor
Drink 2 drops in water or capsule daily.

Food Poisoning
Drink 2 drops in water or capsule as needed.

Rashes
Apply diluted to affected area.

Muscle Aches
Take a drop in a capsule, or massage with carrier oil into affected areas.

Cooking
Use a toothpick to add desired flavor to dishes.

Key Properties
Digestive
Antispasmodic
Analgesic
Antioxidant
Antibacterial

Other Uses
Alzheimer's Disease, Itchy Skin, Joint Pain, Low Energy, Measles, Muscle Tone, Muscle Spasms, Nausea, Neuropathy, Stiffness, Whiplash

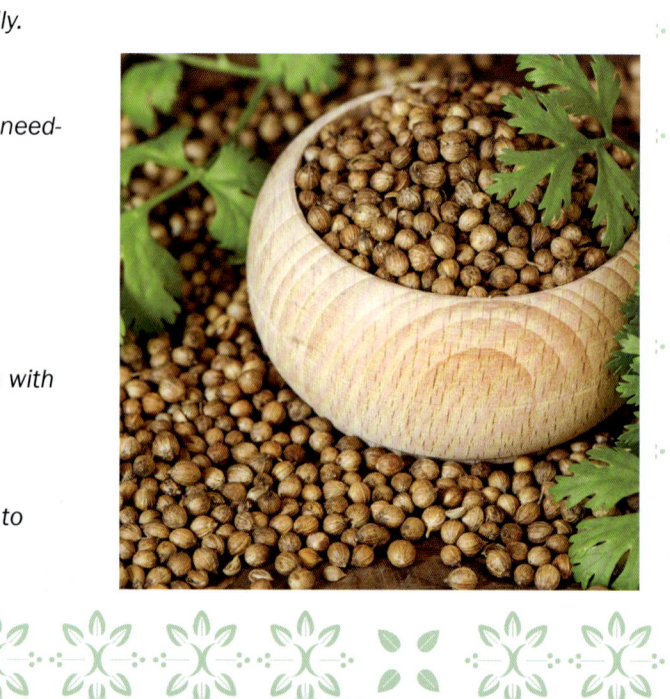

Cypress
Cupressus Sempervirens

Top Uses

Bladder & Urinary Infection
Massage 2 drops over bladder every 2 hours as needed.

Poor Circulation
Apply 2 drops to bottoms of feet morning and evening.

Bone Spurs
Apply 2-4 drops directly onto affected area.

Restless Leg Syndrome
Massage 2 drops with carrier oil into bottoms of feet, calves, and upper legs.

Concussion
Massage 1-3 drops into back of neck, back of skull, and shoulders.

Bed Wetting
Apply 2 drops neat over bladder before bedtime.

Prostate Issues
Massage 1-3 drops over lower abdomen and prostate reflex point.

Application
A T

Safety
Dilute for sensitive skin. Use with caution during pregnancy.

Key Properties
Anti-rheumatic
Antibacterial
Vasoconstrictor
Tonifying
Antiseptic

Other Uses
Aneurysm, Bunions, Edema, Hemorrhoids, Flu, Incontinence, Lou Gehrig's Disease, Ovary Issues, Raynaud's Disease, Tuberculosis, Varicose Veins, Whooping Cough

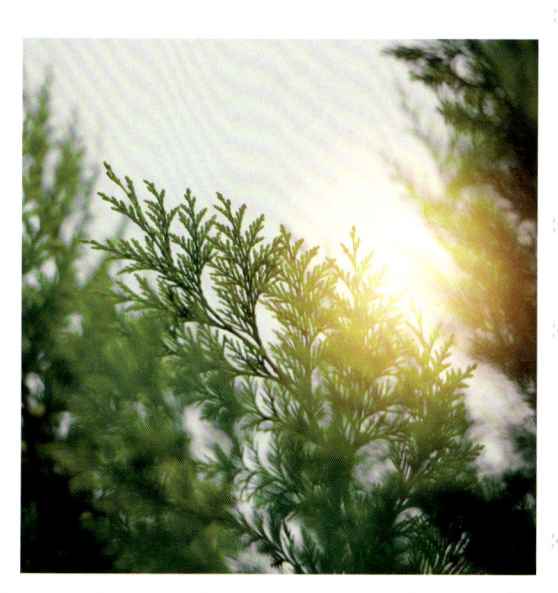

Eucalyptus
Eucalyptus Globulus/Radiata

Top Uses

Bronchitis & Pneumonia
Apply 2-4 drops to chest & mid-back. Also diffuse several drops.

Congestion & Cough
Apply 2-4 drops to chest, and inhale from cupped hands.

Sinusitis
Apply heavily diluted over sinuses, carefully avoiding the eyes.

Asthma
Inhale 2 drops from cupped hands, and apply to lung reflex points.

Mental Fatigue
Inhale 1-2 drops from cupped hands, or diffuse several drops.

Menstrual Cramping
Rub 1-2 drops with carrier oil over abdomen every couple of hours.

Application

Key Properties
Expectorant
Hypotensive
Disinfectant
Antibacterial
Analgesic

Other Uses
Colds, Fever, Flu, Headache, Earache, Insect Bites & Stings, Kidney Stones, Muscle Aches, Neuralgia, Rheumatism, Rhinitis

Safety
Not for use topically on newborns. Eucalyptus Globulus is safe for internal use.

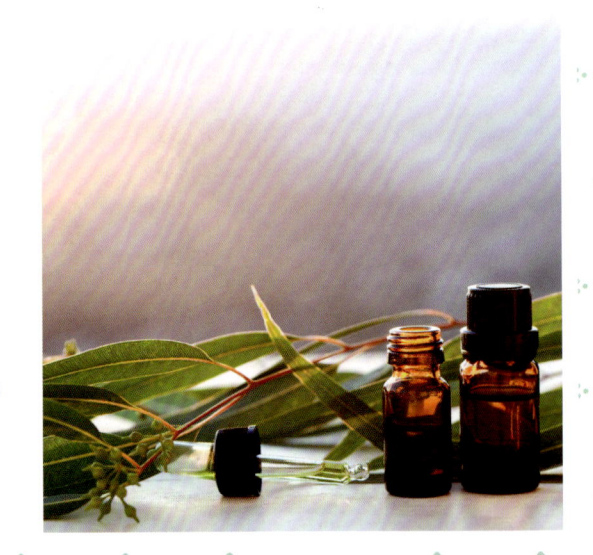

Fennel (sweet)
Foeniculum Vulgare

Top Uses

Digestive Disorders
Drink 1-2 drops in water or a capsule.

Flatulence
Rub 1-2 drops over stomach, or drink with water.

Milk Supply (low)
Massage 1 drop diluted around nipples 2-3 times daily.

Colic
Rub a drop heavily diluted over baby's stomach.

Nausea
Rub 1-2 drops over stomach, or drink a drop in water.

Menstrual Discomfort
Rub a drop over abdomen.

Parasites
Drink 2-4 drops in a capsule 3 times daily.

Application

Safety
Use with caution during pregnancy. Avoid if epileptic.

Key Properties
Emmenagogue
Galactagogue
Mucolytic
Digestive Stimulant
Diuretic

Other Uses
Blood Sugar Imbalance, Constipation, Digestive Disorders, Edema, Fertility Issues, Fluid Retention, Intestinal Parasites, Menopause, PMS, Spasms, Stroke

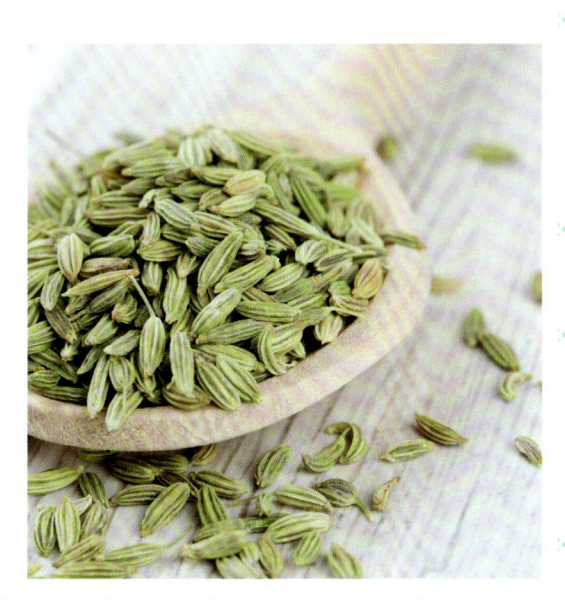

Frankincense

Boswellia Carterii/Frereana

Top Uses

Cellular Health & Function
Take 1-2 drops in a capsule as a daily supplement.

Depression & Anxiety
Use a drop under the tongue, apply to pulse points, or diffuse.

Alzheimer's & Dementia
Apply 2 drops to bottoms of feet and base of skull 2-3 times daily.

Pain & Inflammation
Use a drop under the tongue, or massage into inflamed areas.

Parkinson's Disease
Apply 1-2 drops to brain reflex points and base of skull, and diffuse daily.

Cancer
Take 2-4 drops in a capsule, and apply close to the affected area several times daily. Also diffuse for emotional support.

Application
A T I

Safety
Safe for neat application.

Key Properties
Anticancer
Anti-inflammatory
Antidepressant
Immunostimulant
Restorative

Other Uses
ADHD, Aneurysm, Asthma, Balance, Brain Health, Coma, Concussion, Fibroids, Genital Warts, Immune Support, Lou Gehrig's Disease, Memory, Moles, MRSA, Multiple Sclerosis, Scarring, Sciatica, Warts, Wrinkles

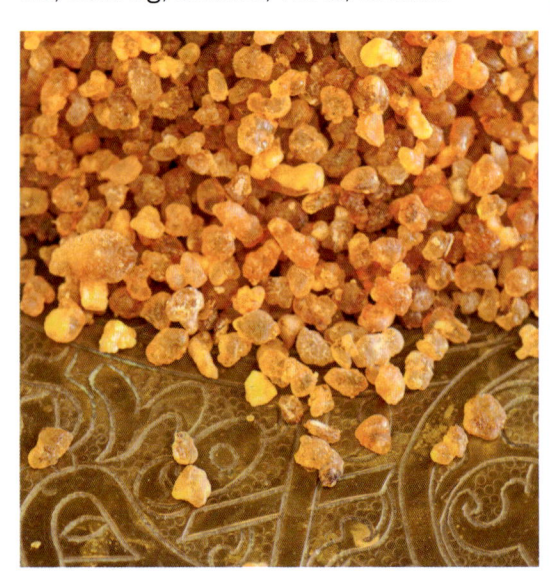

Geranium
Pelargonium Graveolens

Top Uses

Kidney & Liver Support
Rub 1-3 drops directly over liver and kidneys.

Autism
Apply 1-2 drops to the bottoms of feet. Also diffuse daily.

PMS & Hormone Balancing
Apply a drop to pulse points.

Jaundice
Apply 1 drop diluted to bottoms of feet, and diffuse several drops.

Hemorrhoids
Apply heavily diluted to affected areas.

Reproductive Disorders
Apply 1-2 drops to reproductive reflex points, and also over lower abdomen.

Varicose Veins
Massage 1-3 drops diluted into affected areas.

Application

Safety
Dilute for sensitive skin.

Key Properties
Detoxifier
Anti-allergenic
Haemostatic
Regenerative
Anti-toxic

Other Uses
Bleeding, Circulation, Depression, Diarrhea, Gastric Ulcers, Hernia, Low Libido, Menstrual Cramps, Menopause, Neuralgia, Raynaud's Disease, Spasms, Vertigo

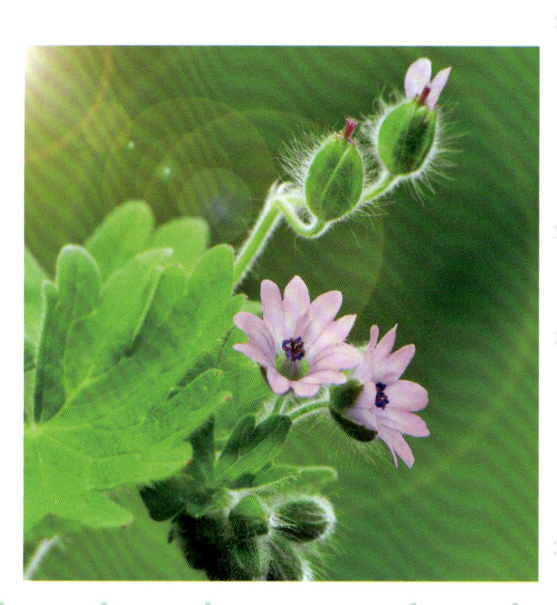

Single Oils

German Chamomile
Matricaria Recutita

Application

Safety
Safe for neat application.

Top Uses

Eczema & Psoriasis
Apply 1-2 drops diluted to affected areas several times a day.

Arthritis
Massage 1-2 drops neat into affected areas.

Allergies
Inhale 1-2 drops from cupped hands, or diffuse several drops. Also rub a small amount over sinuses, carefully avoiding eyes.

Acne & Pimples
Put a dab onto problematic areas.

Menstrual Cramping & Mood
Massage 1-2 drops onto lower abdomen, and inhale from cupped hands.

Sleep Issues
Rub 1-2 drops onto temples and bottoms of feet. Also diffuse next to bedside.

Motion Sickness & Nausea
Inhale 1-2 drops from cupped hands, or rub onto stomach.

Key Properties
Anti-inflammatory
Emmenagogue
Analgesic
Calming
Stomachic

Other Uses
Allergies, Anxiety, Chilblains, Depression, Detox, Endometriosis, Inflammation, Rashes, Respiratory Conditions, Rheumatism, Stomachache, Stress, Wounds

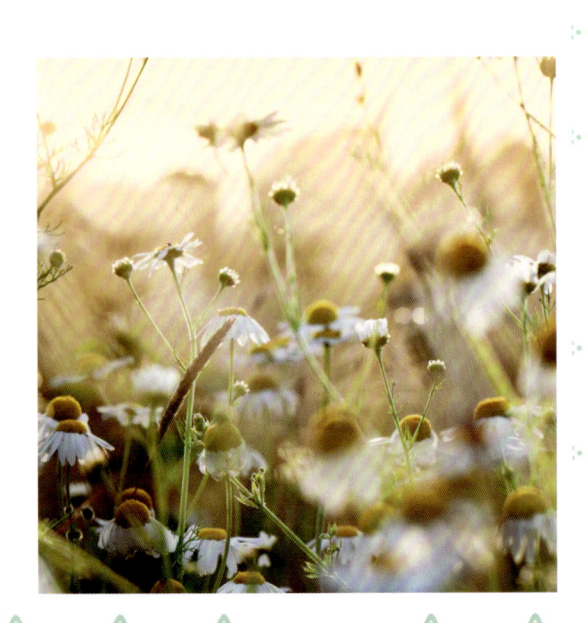

Ginger
Zingiber Officinale

Top Uses

Upset Stomach & Nausea
Drink 1-2 drops in water or a capsule.

Vomiting
Rub a drop diluted over stomach.

Constipation
Apply 1-2 drops diluted over stomach, or take in a capsule.

Congestion & Cough
Diffuse several drops, or apply 1-3 drops diluted over chest.

Immune Support
Apply 1-3 drops to bottoms of feet, or take in a capsule.

Cold & Flu
Apply 1-3 drops to bottoms of feet, or drink in a capsule.

Cooking
Use a toothpick to achieve desired flavor.

Application
A, T, I

Safety
Dilute for sensitive skin.

Key Properties
Stimulant
Decongestant
Anti-inflammatory
Digestive
Neurotonic

Other Uses
Aneurysm, Breast Enlargement, Cholesterol, Convulsions, Endometriosis, Epilepsy, Fragile Hair, Hot Flashes, Impotence, Lactation, Parkinson's, Premenopause, Seizures

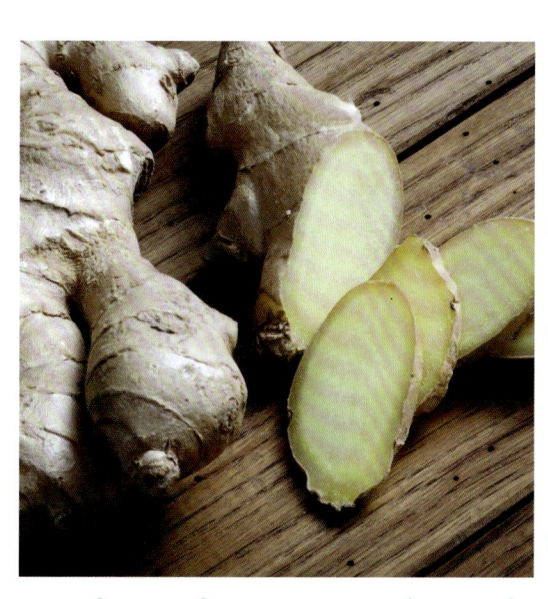

Grapefruit
Citrus X Paradisi

Top Uses

Weight Loss
Apply 10 drops diluted with carrier oil over cellulite and other fatty areas.

Detox
Drink 1-3 drops in water a few times a day for several days.

Smoking Addiction
Drink 1-3 drops in water after meals to cleanse the palate.

Appetite Suppressant
Diffuse several drops, or drink 1-3 drops in water.

Antiviral Support
Apply 1-2 drops to bottoms of feet, or drink in water.

Gallbladder Stones
Drink 1-3 drops in water 3 times daily.

Application

Safety
Avoid UV exposure for 12 hours after topical use.

Key Properties
Antioxidant
Astringent
Expectorant
Diuretic
Antiseptic

Other Uses
Anorexia, Bulimia, Dry Throat, Edema, Energy, Hangovers, Jet Lag, Lymphatic Congestion, Miscarriage Recovery, Obesity, Overeating

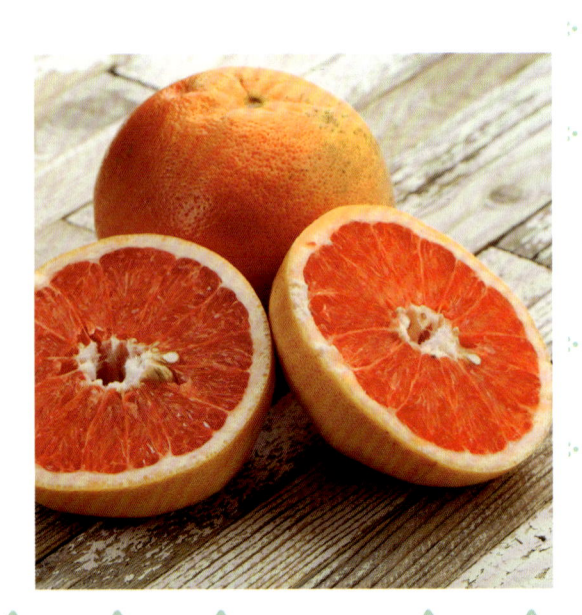

Helichrysum
Helichrysum Italicum

Top Uses

Bleeding
Apply to clean wound to stop bleeding.

Cuts & Scrapes
Apply neat or diluted to help wounds heal without scarring.

Eczema & Psoriasis
Apply 1-2 drops diluted to affected areas a few times daily.

Tinnitus
Apply a drop behind ear.

Shock
Diffuse 3-6 drops, or massage a drop into neck and shoulders.

Cholesterol
Take 1-3 drops in a capsule, and apply to bottoms of feet.

Viral Infections
Take 1-2 drops in a capsule, or diffuse.

Application
A T I

Safety
Safe for neat application.

Key Properties
Anticatarrhal
Neuroprotective
Nervine
Analgesic
Antispasmodic

Other Uses
AIDS/HIV, Broken Blood Vessels, Bruises, Cuts, Earache, Fibroids, Gallbladder Infections, Hemorrhaging, Hernias, Herpes, Lymphatic Drainage, Nose Bleed, Sciatica, Staph Infection, Stretch Marks, Wrinkles

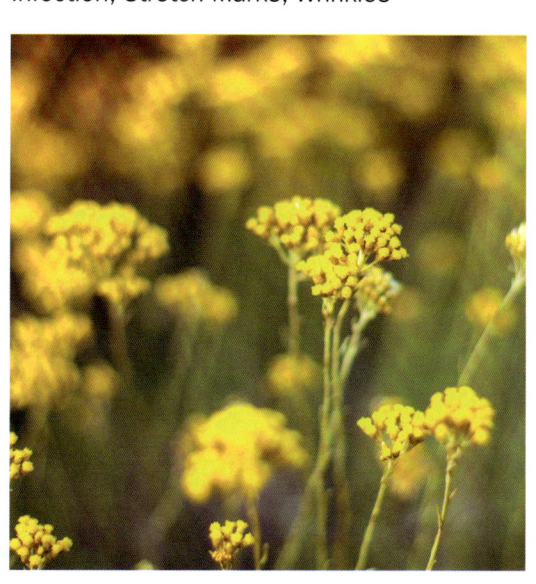

Single Oils

Juniper Berry
Juniperus Communis

Top Uses

Diabetes
Take 1-2 drops in a capsule daily. Combine with Cinnamon and Coriander.

Kidney Detox & Infections
Rub 1-2 drops over kidneys, or take in a capsule.

Kidney Stones
Apply 1-2 drops over kidneys.

High Cholesterol
Take 1-2 drops in a capsule, and apply to bottoms of feet.

Tinnitus
Apply a drop behind affected ear.

Chronic Fatigue
Massage 1-2 drops over adrenals and onto pulse points, and diffuse.

Urinary Tract Infection
Apply 2-4 drops over bladder.

Application

Safety
Safe for neat application.

Key Properties
Anti-rheumatic
Carminative
Anti-parasitic
Diuretic
Antiseptic

Other Uses
Acne, Anxiety, Bacteria, Bloating, Cellulite, Cystitis, Detoxifying, Fluid Retention, Heavy Legs, Jaundice, Menstrual Cramping, Mental Exhaustion, Stress, Ulcers, Viruses

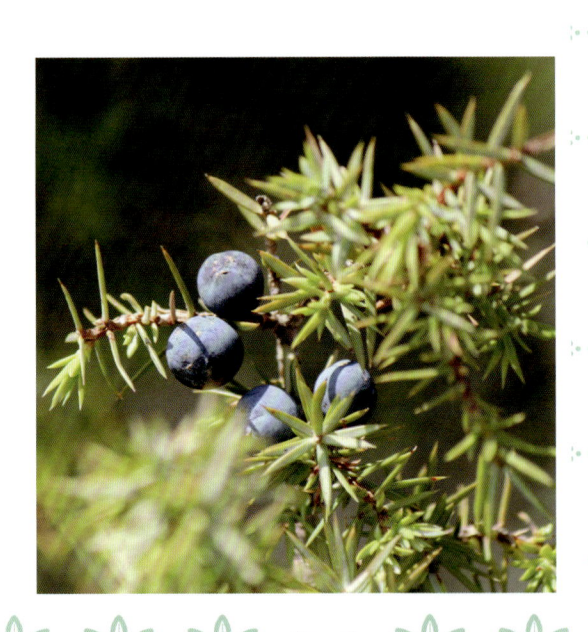

Lavender (true)
Lavandula Angustifolia

Top Uses

Sleep Issues
Apply 2 drops to bottoms of feet and temples, or diffuse near bedside.

Stress & Anxiety
Apply 1-2 drops to temples, or diffuse several drops.

Headaches & Migraines
Apply 1-2 drops to temples and base of skull.

Skin Irritations & Burns
Apply 1-3 drops neat or diluted to affected areas.

Allergies & Hay Fever
Put a drop under tongue for 30 seconds, then swallow with water.

Cuts, Blisters, & Scrapes
Apply neat or diluted to affected areas.

Irritability
Apply 1-2 drops to pulse points.

Application
A T I

Safety
Safe for neat application.

Key Properties
Antihistamine
Sedative
Cytophylactic
Hypotensive
Antispasmodic

Other Uses
Allergies, Bites, Blisters, Chicken Pox, Club Foot, Colic, Convulsions, Crying, Dandruff, Diaper Rash, Gangrene, Giardia, Impetigo, Insomnia, Poison Ivy & Oak, Seizures, Stings, Tachycardia, Teething Pain, Ticks

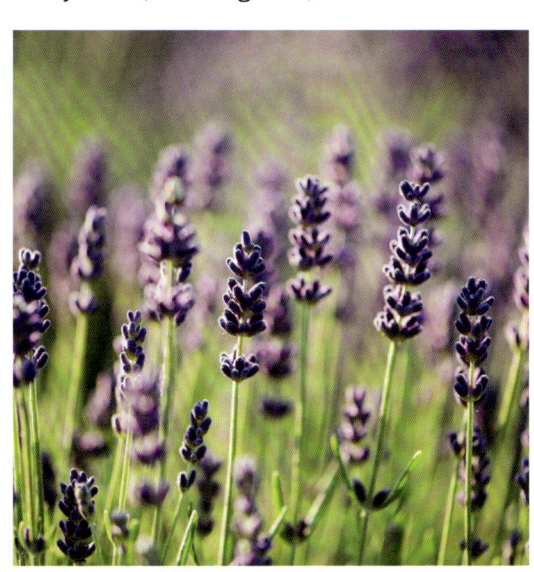

Single Oils

Lemon
Citrus Limon

Top Uses

Detox
Drink 1-3 drops in water a few times a day for several days. Also apply to bottoms of feet.

Energy
Drink 1-3 drops in water, or inhale from cupped hands.

Permanent Marker
Rub several drops with a clean rag.

Sore Throat
Take 1-2 drops with a spoonful of honey.

Household Cleaner
Use several drops with water in a glass spray bottle. Add vinegar if desired.

Food & Cooking
Use in smoothies, juices, and dressings.

Increase Alkalinity
Drink 1-3 drops in water.

Application

Safety
Avoid UV exposure 12 hours after topical application.

Key Properties
Antibacterial
Antiseptic
Disinfectant
Mucolytic
Diuretic

Other Uses
Anxiety, Cold Sores, Colds, Concentration, Constipation, Depression, Disinfectant, Dysentery, Flu, Furniture Polish, Greasy Hair, High Blood Pressure, Kidney Stones, MRSA, Pancreatitis, Parasites, Tonsillitis

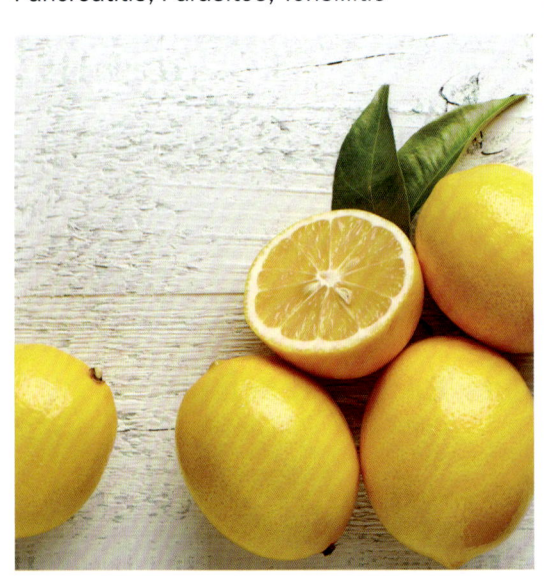

Lemongrass
Cymbopogon Flexuosus

Top Uses

High Cholesterol
Take 1-2 drops in capsule.

Thyroid Support (hypo & hyper)
Apply a drop diluted over thyroid.

Ligament & Tendon Injuries
Apply 1-2 drops diluted to painful areas.

Stomach Ulcers
Take 1 drop in a capsule with 1 drop Frankincense a few times a day for a few days.

Lactose Intolerance
Take 1 drop in a capsule.

Immune Support
Apply 1-3 drops to bottoms of feet.

Cooking
Use toothpick to achieve desired flavor.

Application
A T I

Key Properties
Antimicrobial
Anti-inflammatory
Anti-carcinoma
Anti-mutagenic
Decongestant

Safety
Dilute for sensitive skin. Do not use internally for more than 10 days.

Other Uses
Airborne Bacteria, Bladder Infection, Carpal Tunnel, Charley Horses, Connective Tissue Injury, Constipation, Frozen Shoulder, Lymphatic Drainage, Paralysis, Sprains, Urinary Tract infection

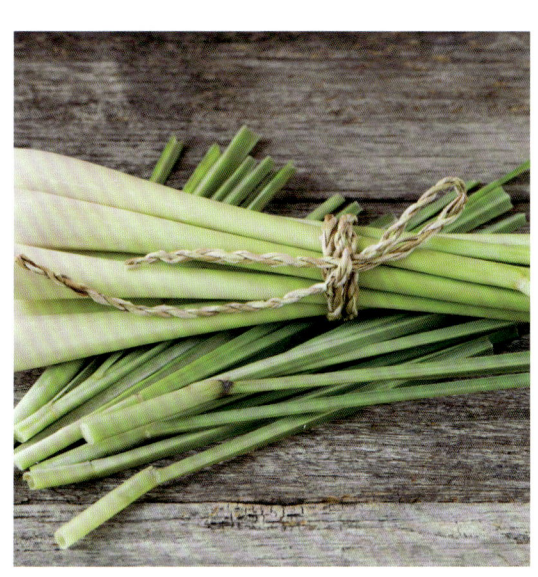

Lime
Citrus Aurantifolia

Top Uses

Cold & Flu
Drink 1-3 drops in water, and also diffuse several drops.

Chronic Cough
Apply 2-4 drops over chest, mid-back, and lung reflex points.

Sore Throat
Gargle 2 drops with water, or add a drop to hot tea.

Antioxidant
Drink 1-3 drops in water.

Cold Sores
Apply 1 drop diluted to affected area.

Mental Clarity
Diffuse several drops, or inhale from cupped hands.

Bacterial Infections
Apply 1-2 drops diluted to affected area.

Application
A T I

Safety
Avoid UV exposure for 12 hours after topical application.

Key Properties
Antiseptic
Antioxidant
Antibacterial
Tonic
Anti-inflammatory

Other Uses
Antiviral Support, Blood Pressure, Cellulite, Depression, Detox, Energy, Exhaustion, Fever, Gallstones, Gum Removal, Herpes, Memory, Water Purification

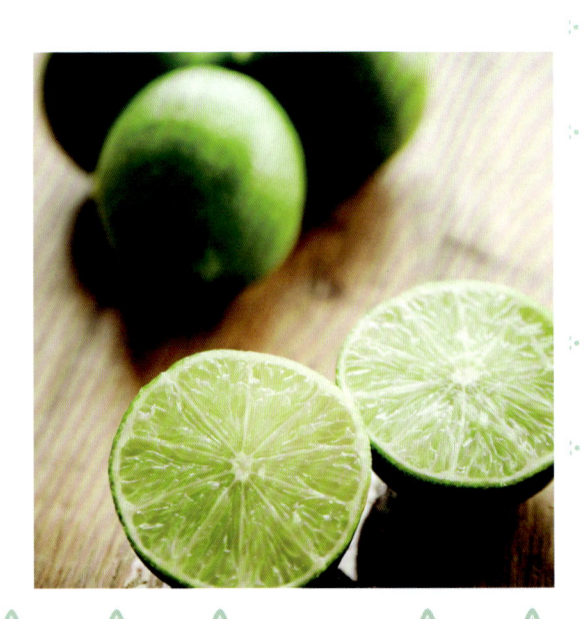

Marjoram
Origanum Majorana

Top Uses

High Blood Pressure
Apply 2 drops to bottoms of feet, or take in a capsule.

Carpal Tunnel & Arthritis
Massage 1-2 drops into affected areas.

Muscle Injury
Massage 2 drops diluted into injured muscles.

Irritable Bowel Syndrome
Take 1-2 drops in a capsule, or rub clockwise over abdomen.

Diverticulitis
Take 1-2 drops in a capsule daily.

Chronic Stress
Massage 1-2 drops onto back of neck.

Pancreatitis
Apply 1-2 drops neat over pancreas area.

Application
A T I

Safety
Use with caution during beginning of pregnancy.

Key Properties
Digestive Stimulant
Hypotensive
Sedative
Vasodilator
Antispasmodic

Other Uses
Arterial Vasodilator, Bruises, Colic, Constipation, Croup, Headache, Gastrointestinal Disorders, Insomnia, Menstrual Problems, Parkinson's, Prolapsed Mitral Valve, Ringworm, Sprains, Whiplash

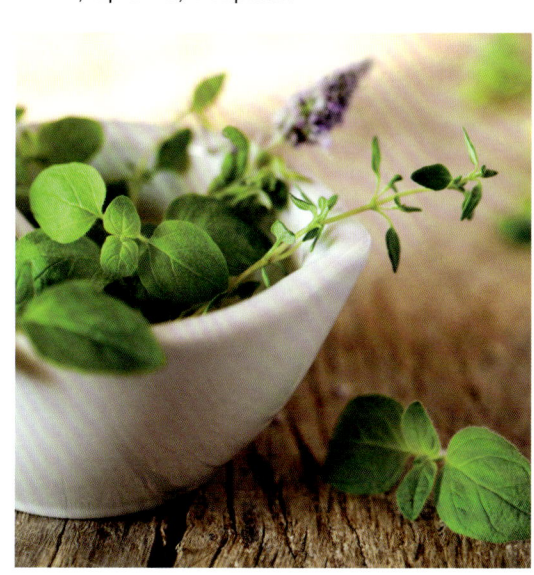

Myrrh
Commiphora Myrrha

Top Uses

Thyroid Support
Rub 1-2 drops over thyroid.

Wrinkles & Fine Lines
Massage 1-2 drops into needed areas as desired, or add to facial moisturizer.

Gum Disease
Apply 1-2 drops to gums, or swish with water as a mouth rinse.

Mucus & Bronchitis
Apply 1-2 drops to chest, or diffuse.

Nail Fungus
Apply a drop directly to affected nail.

Anxiety & Depression
Inhale 1-2 drops from cupped hands, or diffuse a few drops.

Eczema & Skin Infections
Apply 1-2 drops diluted to affected areas.

Application

Safety
Use with caution during pregnancy.

Key Properties
Expectorant
Carminative
Anti-inflammatory
Antimicrobial
Antiviral

Other Uses
Cancer, Chapped Skin, Congestion, Dysentery, Gum Bleeding, Hepatitis, Liver Cirrhosis, Scabies, Stretch Marks

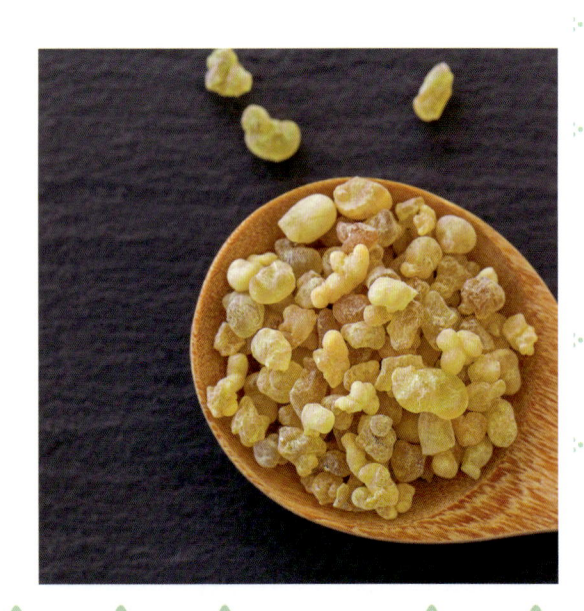

Myrtle
Myrtus Communis

Top Uses

Sinus Infection
Apply a drop over sinuses, carefully avoiding the eyes. Also use a drop in a netty pot.

Bronchitis & Cough
Apply 2-4 drops over chest and mid-back, and diffuse several drops.

Cystitis & Urinary Infection
Apply 2-4 drops diluted over bladder.

Impotence
Apply 1-2 drops to wrists and pulse points, and diffuse.

Chronic Fatigue
Apply 1-2 drops over adrenal areas, or wear as perfume or cologne.

Head Lice
Add 1-2 drops into shampoo. Shampoo twice until problem is resolved.

Application

Safety
Use caution during pregnancy and while breast feeding.

Key Properties
Anticatarrhal
Aphrodisiac
Astringent
Expectorant
Regenerative

Other Uses
Acne, Boils, Bronchial Infection, Colds, Emotional Exhaustion, Heavy Legs, Insomnia, Mite Bites, Parasite Infections, Psoriasis, Skin Disorders

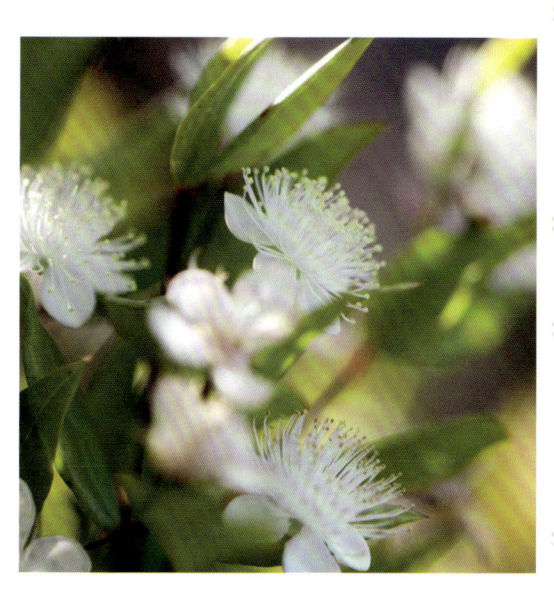

Nutmeg
Myristica Fragrans

Top Uses

Intestinal Spasms
Massage 1-2 drops diluted over stomach and lower abdomen.

Stomach Upset
Rub 1-2 drops over stomach, or take in a capsule.

Muscle Aches & Cramps
Massage 2-4 drops neat or diluted into affected muscles.

Menstrual Cramping
Rub 1-2 drops over lower abdomen and reproductive reflex points.

Insomnia & Restlessness
Put a drop under the tongue 30 minutes before bedtime, or diffuse next to bedside.

Nervous Tension
Rub a drop into temples, apply to bottoms of feet, or diffuse.

Application
A T I

Safety
Use caution during pregnancy.

Key Properties
Analgesic
Anti-infectious
Antiseptic
Digestive Stimulant
Nervine

Other Uses
Arthritis, Circulation, Congestion, Cooking, Depression, Halitosis, Hormone Balance, Inflammation, Liver Detox, Kidney Infection & Disease, Mood Swings, Muscle Injury, Nausea, Rheumatism

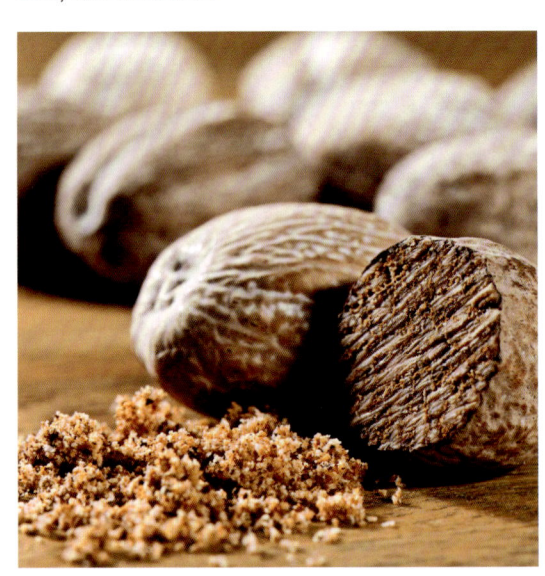

Orange
Citrus Sinensis

Top Uses

Cheering & Mood Enhancement
Inhale 1-2 drops from cupped hands, or diffuse several drops.

Sleep Issues
Put a drop under tongue 30 minutes before bedtime.

Low Energy
Drink 1-3 drops in water, or inhale from cupped hands.

Anxiety & Depression
Inhale 1-2 drops from cupped hands, or diffuse several drops.

Immune Support
Gargle 2 drops with water, or apply to bottoms of feet.

Smoothies, Dressings, & Sauces
Add according to taste.

Application
A, T, I

Safety
Avoid UV exposure 12 hours after topical application.

Key Properties
Antiseptic
Carminative
Antidepressant
Immunostimulant
Anti-carcinoma

Other Uses
Cellulite, Colds, Creativity, Depression, Detox, Fear, Fluid Retention, Heart Palpitations, Insomnia, Menopause, Nervousness, Scurvy, Sluggish Digestion, Withdrawal Issues

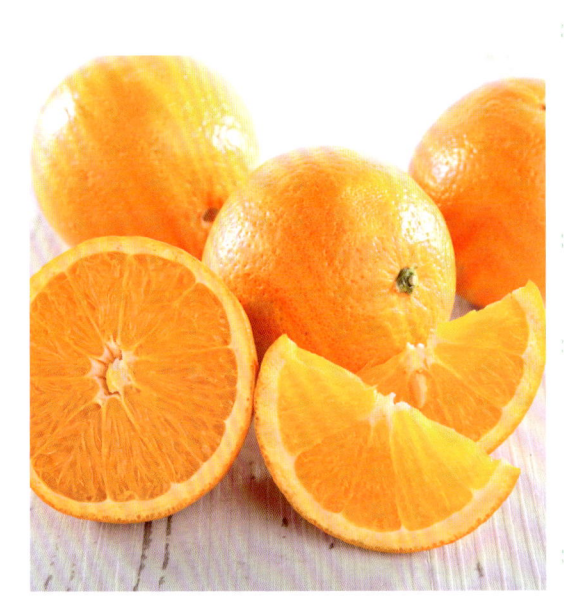

Oregano
Origanum Vulgare

Top Uses

Bacterial & Viral Infection
Take 2-4 drops in a capsule for internal issues.

Candida & Staph Infection
Take 1-3 drops in a capsule for 7-10 days.

Warts
Apply a dab directly to wart with toothpick, avoiding surrounding skin.

Rheumatoid Arthritis
Massage 1 drop heavily diluted into affected area. Also take in a capsule.

Strep Throat & Tonsillitis
Gargle a drop in water. Also take 1-3 drops in a capsule.

Pneumonia & Whooping Cough
Diffuse 1-3 drops, sitting nearby the diffuser for a few minutes. Also rub onto bottoms of feet.

Application

Key Properties
Antibacterial
Antiviral
Anti-fungal
Anti-parasitic
Immunostimulant

Other Uses
Athlete's Foot, Calluses, Canker Sores, Carpal Tunnel, Control Issues, Ebola, Fungal Infections, Intestinal Parasites, MRSA, Nasal Polyps, Plague, Ringworm

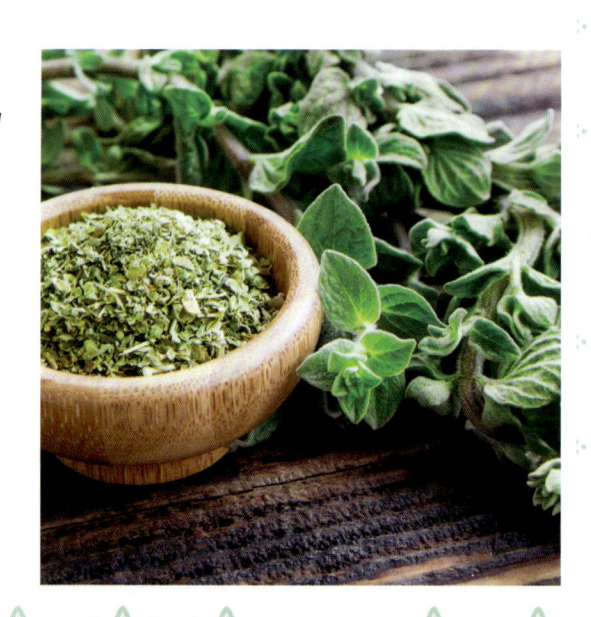

Safety
Dilute heavily for topical use. Do not use internally more than 10 days in a row.

Patchouli
Pogostemon Cablin

Top Uses

Shingles
Take 1-3 drops in a capsule, and apply to bottoms of feet.

Diuretic
Apply 1-2 drops to lower abdomen.

Wrinkle Prevention
Add a drop to daily facial toner or moisturizer.

Weight Loss
Take 1-2 drops in a capsule with other weight loss essential oils.

Dopamine Shortage
Diffuse 2-4 drops, or apply to pulse points.

Dandruff
Massage 1-2 drops with carrier oil into clean, dry scalp after showering at night.

Herpes
Apply a drop neat to affected areas.

Application

Safety
Safe for neat application.

Key Properties
Antidepressant
Aphrodisiac
Sedative
Antispasmodic
Insecticide

Other Uses
Abscess, Cellulite, Chapped Skin, Depression, Dermatitis, Hemorrhoids, Hives, Irritability, Mastitis, Parasitic Skin Infection, PMS, Weeping Wounds

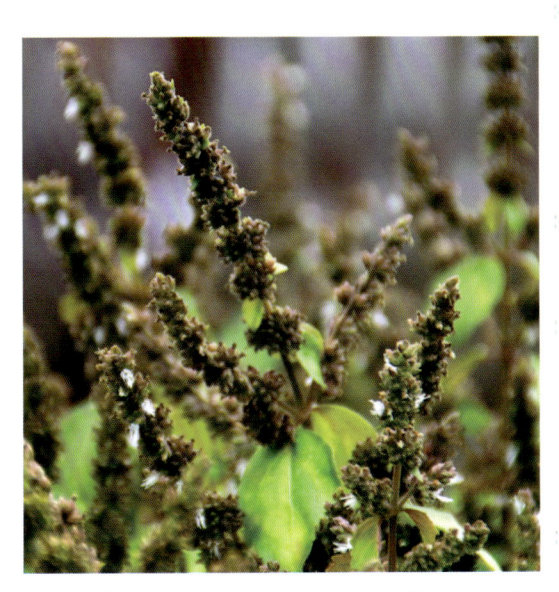

Peppermint
Mentha Piperita

Application

Safety
Dilute for sensitive skin.

Top Uses

Digestive Upset
Drink 1-2 drops in water, or massage directly over stomach.

Headache & Migraine
Massage 1-2 drops into temples and base of skull, avoiding eyes.

Fever
Apply 1-2 drops to back of neck, or add to a cool, wet rag.

Asthma & Cough
Apply 1-3 drops diluted over chest and lung reflex points. Also diffuse several drops.

Bad Breath
Lick a dab from your fingertip.

Low Energy & Mental Fatigue
Drink 1-2 drops in water, or diffuse.

Muscle & Joint Pain
Rub a drop diluted into affected areas.

Key Properties
Stimulating
Anti-inflammatory
Analgesic
Antispasmodic
Expectorant

Other Uses
Alertness, Allergies, Autism, Burns, Cravings, Gastritis, Hangover, Hot Flashes, Hypothyroidism, Loss of Sense of Smell, Memory, Milk Supply (decrease), Osteoporosis, Sciatica, Sinusitis, Typhoid

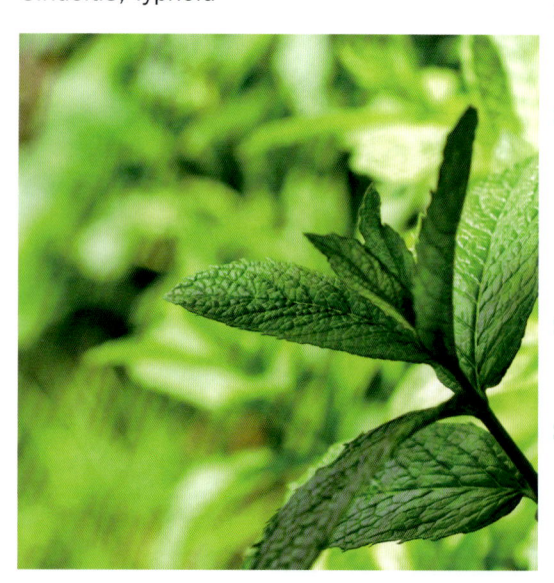

Roman Chamomile
Chamaemelum Nobile

Application: A, T, I

Safety
Safe for neat application.

Top Uses

Sleep Issues & Insomnia
Apply 1-2 drops to temples and wrists, or diffuse next to bedside.

Diaper Rash
Apply a drop heavily diluted with carrier oil to baby's skin.

Panic Attacks
Carry on person, and breathe a drop deeply from cupped hands as needed.

Parasites & Worms
Apply 1-2 drops over abdomen, and take 2-4 drops in a capsule three times daily.

Crying
Add a drop to front of shirt or sleeve, and also diffuse a few drops.

PMS & Cramps
Apply a drop over abdomen, or use in massage over lower back.

Key Properties
Antihistamine
Sedative
Antibacterial
Immunostimulant
Anti-fungal

Other Uses
Allergies, Anorexia, Bee/Hornet Sting, Club Foot, Dysentery, Hyperactivity, Menopause, Muscle Spasms, Neuralgia, Rashes, Shock, Sore Nipples (breast feeding)

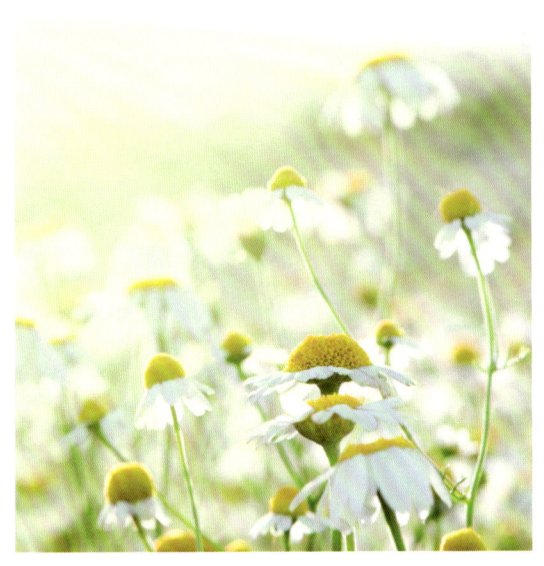

Rosemary
Rosmarinus Officinalis

Top Uses

Mental & Adrenal Fatigue
Inhale 1-2 drops from cupped hands, or take in a capsule.

Chronic Cough
Apply 2-4 drops to lung reflex points, over chest, and over mid-back. Also diffuse.

Hair Loss
Work 2 drops into scalp before washing with shampoo.

Focus & Memory Issues
Apply a drop over forehead, or diffuse a few drops.

Cold & Flu
Apply 1-2 drops diluted over chest.

Low Blood Pressure
Massage with carrier oil into legs and bottles of feet.

Jet Lag
Apply 1-2 drops to temples after flying.

Application

Safety
Avoid during pregnancy, if epileptic, or with high blood pressure.

Key Properties
Anticatarrhal
Immunostimulant
Anti-carcinoma
Anti-mutagenic
Steroidal

Other Uses
Alcohol Addiction, Adenitis, Arthritis, Bell's Palsy, Cellulite, Club Foot, Constipation, Headaches, Kidney Infection, Lice, Muscular Dystrophy, Osteoarthritis, Schmidt's Syndrome, Sinusitis

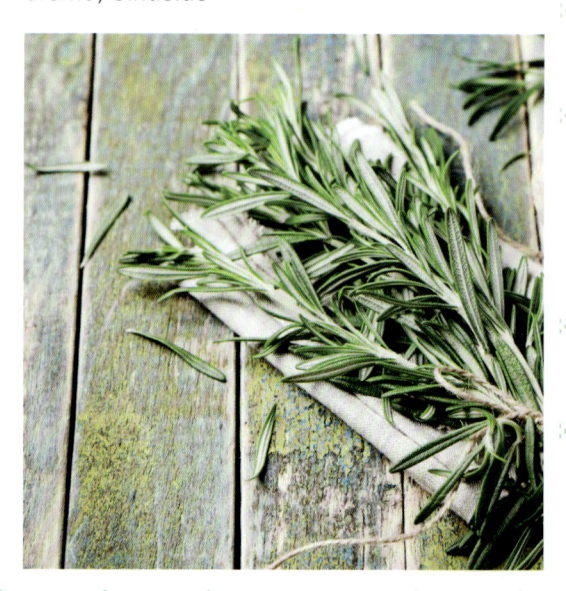

Sandalwood
Santalum Austrocaledonicum

Top Uses

Rashes & Skin Conditions
Apply 1-2 drops diluted to affected areas.

Meditation
Apply a drop to temples or pulse points, or diffuse several drops to enhance meditation.

Alzheimer's Disease
Apply 1-2 drops to the base of skull, or take 1-3 drops in a capsule a few times daily.

Cancer & Tumors
Take 1-2 drops in a capsule, apply directly to affected areas, or diffuse several drops.

Low Testosterone
Take 1-2 drops in a capsule, or apply to pulse points and lower abdomen.

Scars
Massage 1-2 drops into scars often.

Dry Scalp
Massage 1-2 drops into scalp before or after shampooing.

Application

Safety
Safe for neat application.

Key Properties
Anti-carcinoma
Anti-inflammatory
Astringent
Calming
Antidepressant

Other Uses
Aphrodisiac, Back Pain, Blemishes, Calming, Cartilage Repair, Coma, Dry Skin, Exhaustion, Hiccups, Laryngitis, Lou Gehrig's Disease, Moles, Multiple Sclerosis, UV radiation, Yoga

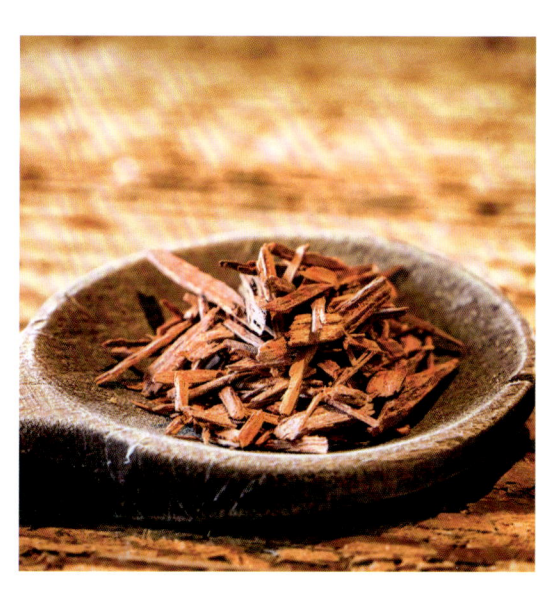

Scotch Pine
Pinus Sylvestris

Top Uses

Muscle Pain & Fatigue
Massage 2-4 drops with carrier oil into affected muscles.

Rheumatism & Gout
Rub 1-2 drops into affected areas, and onto bottoms of feet.

Fatigue & Exhaustion
Inhale 1-2 drops from cupped hands, or diffuse several drops.

Urinary Infection
Rub 1-2 drops over lower abdomen.

Respiratory Conditions
Rub 2-4 drops onto chest and mid-back, or diffuse several drops.

Sinus Congestion
Inhale 1-2 drops from cupped hands. Carefully apply around sinuses, avoiding eyes.

Cold & Flu
Rub 1-3 drops onto bottoms of feet, and diffuse several drops.

Application

Safety
Dilute for sensitive skin.

Key Properties
Anti-microbial
Decongestant
Diuretic
Expectorant
Tonic

Other Uses
Arthritis, Bronchial Infection, Dermatitis, Fleas, Infections, Joint Pain, Ligament Injury, Metabolism Boost, Muscle Injury, Nervous Exhaustion, PTSD, Scabies

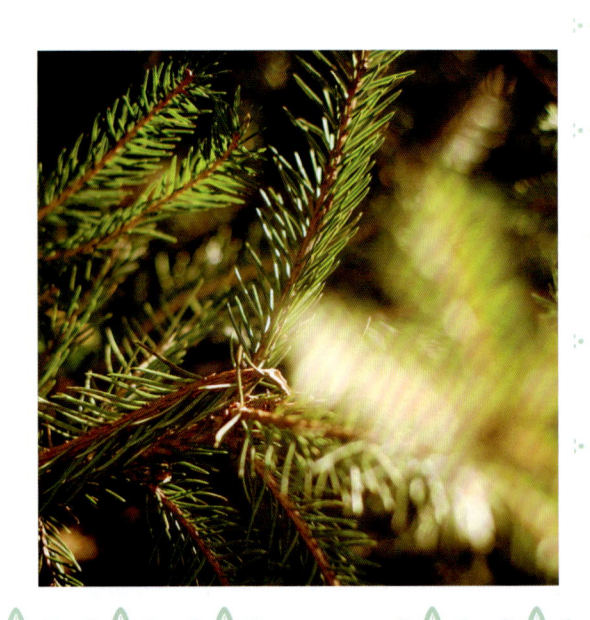

Spearmint
Mentha Spicata

Top Uses

Colic
Apply a drop heavily diluted to baby's stomach.

Indigestion
Drink 1-2 drops in water or in a capsule.

Nausea
Inhale 1-2 drops from cupped hands, or rub over stomach.

Muscle Aches
Massage 1-2 drops diluted into achy muscles, or add to hot bath.

Bad Breath
Swish 1-2 drops in water as a mouthwash.

Heavy Menstruation
Apply 1-2 drops over back of neck and abdomen during period.

Cooking & Cocktails
Add a toothpick swirl to achieve desired flavor.

Application

Safety
Safe for neat application.

Key Properties
Stimulant
Antiseptic
Anti-inflammatory
Digestive stimulant
Deodorant

Other Uses
Acne, Bronchitis, Headaches, Focus, Migraines, Nervous Fatigue, Respiratory Infections, Sores, Scars

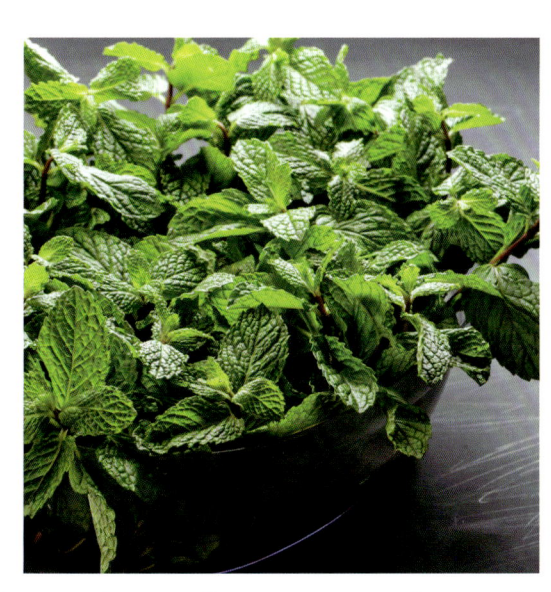

Spruce
Picea Mariana

Top Uses

Headache & Migraines
Massage a drop into temples and base of skull.

Muscle Soreness
Massage 2-4 drops diluted into sore muscles.

Focus & Mental Clarity
Inhale from cupped hands, or diffuse several drops.

Skin Irritations
Apply heavily diluted to irritated skin.

Congestion
Rub 1-2 drops over chest and lung reflex points, or diffuse several drops.

Cough
Inhale 1-2 drops from cupped hands, or rub over chest and mid-back.

Circulation Issues
Apply 1-2 drops to bottoms of feet.

Application

Safety
Safe for neat application.

Key Properties
Anti-arthritic
Analgesic
Antiseptic
Stimulant
Antioxidant

Other Uses
Airborne Pathogens, Arthritis, Asthma, Bursitis, Bruising, Constipation, Depression, Edema, Emotional Congestion, Energy, Generational Patterns, Weight Gain, Sinus Issues

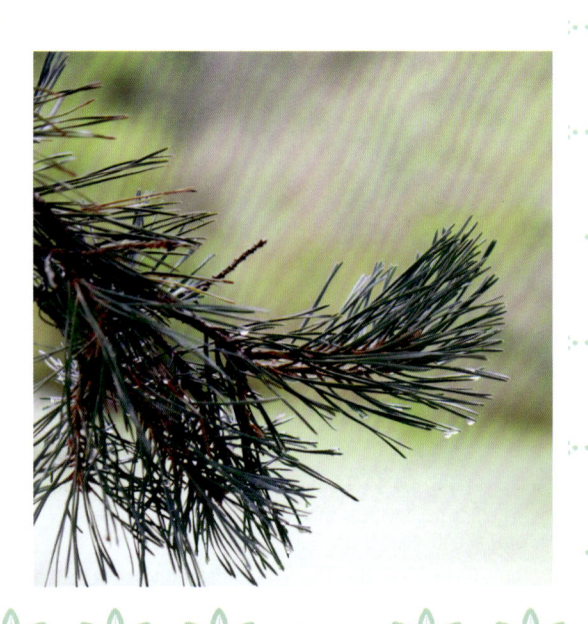

Tangerine
Citrus Reticulata

Top Uses

Nervous Exhaustion
Diffuse 4-8 drops, or wear a drop on pulse points.

Stress-Induced Insomnia
Inhale 1-2 drops during stressful times of the day. Use a drop under the tongue before bedtime.

Flatulence & Constipation
Rub 1-2 drops clockwise over stomach, or drink with water.

Cellulite
Massage several drops with carrier oil into cellulite areas.

Congestion
Rub 2-4 drops over chest and mid-back. Also diffuse several drops.

Discouragement
Inhale 1-2 drops from cupped hands. Also drink 1-3 drops in water.

Application
A T I

Safety
Avoid UV exposure for 12 afters after topical application

Key Properties
Uplifting
Antioxidant
Cytophylactic
Stomachic
Mucolytic

Other Uses
Anxious Feelings, Chronic Fatigue, Circulation, Detox, Digestive Problems, Muscle Aches, Muscle Spasms, Parasites, Water Retention

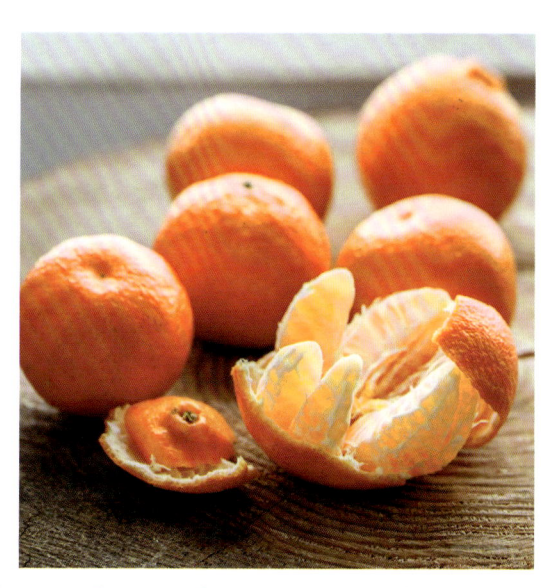

Tea Tree
Melaleuca Alternifolia

Top Uses

Acne & Blemishes
Apply a dab to affected areas.

Herpes
Apply a drop diluted to affected areas.

Rashes & Eczema
Apply 1-2 drops diluted or neat to affected areas.

Dandruff
Add 2 drops to shampoo daily.

Athlete's Foot
Apply 2-4 drops neat to clean, dry feet.

Staph Infections
Take 1-2 drops in a capsule.

Strep Throat & Tonsillitis
Gargle 2 drops with water, and rub 1-2 drops diluted to outside of throat.

Cuts & Wounds
Apply a drop to and around wounded area.

Application

Safety
Dilute for sensitive skin.

Key Properties
Antibacterial
Anti-fungal
Antiseptic
Anti-parasitic
Antiviral

Other Uses
Aneurysm, Bacterial Infections, Cankers, Candida, Cavities, Cold Sores, Dermatitis, Ear infections, Fungal Infections, Hepatitis, Infected Wounds, MRSA, Nail Fungus, Pink Eye, Rubella, Thrush

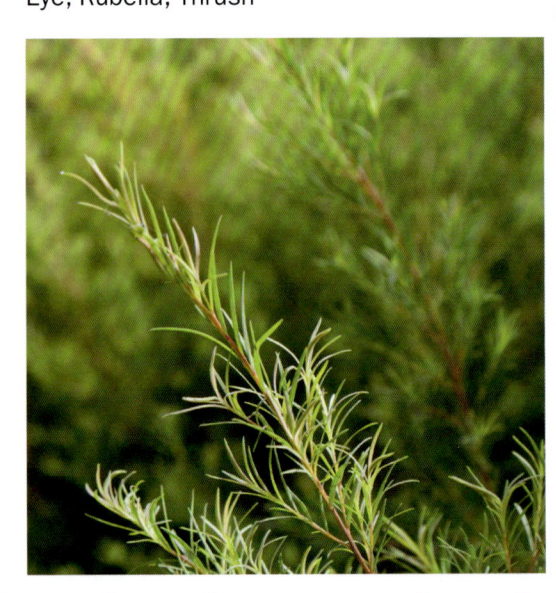

Thyme
Thymus Vulgaris

Top Uses

Cough, Cold, & Flu
Diffuse 1-2 drops, apply to the bottoms of feet, or take in a capsule.

Chronic Fatigue
Take 1-2 drops in a capsule, or apply heavily diluted over adrenal glands. Also use a drop in a hot bath.

Bacterial Infection
Take 1-2 drops in a capsule, or apply to bottoms of feet.

Mononucleosis
Take 2 drops in a capsule 3 times daily. Also apply to the bottoms of feet.

Bronchitis
Apply 1-2 drops heavily diluted over chest and lung reflex points.

Skin Infections
Apply a drop heavily diluted to affected area.

Application

Safety
Use caution during pregnancy, if epileptic, or with high blood pressure.

Key Properties
Antiviral
Analgesic
Mucolytic
Anti-rheumatic
Vermifuge

Other Uses
Antioxidant, Asthma, Bites/Stings, Blood Clots, Croup, Eczema/Dermatitis, Fragile Hair, Fungal Infections, Greasy Hair, hair Loss, Laryngitis, Mold, Numbness, Parasites, Prostatits, Tendinitis, Tuberculosis

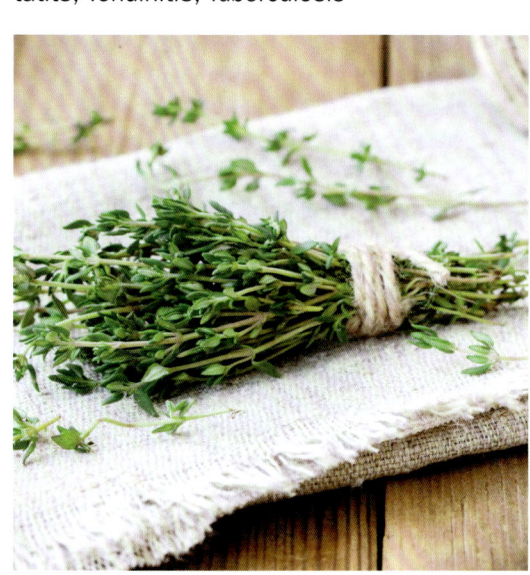

Vetiver
Vetiveria Zizanioides

Top Uses

ADD/ADHD
Apply 1-2 drops behind ears and on the back of the neck.

Neuropathy
Apply 1-2 drops to bottoms of feet and alone spine.

Sleep & Insomnia
Apply 1-2 drops to bottoms of feet and along spine, and diffuse.

PTSD & Anxiety
Apply 1-2 drops behind ears, or diffuse.

Skin Irritation
Apply 1-2 drops diluted to affected areas.

Balance Issues
Apply 1-2 drops behind ears.

Stress-Related Menstrual Issues
Apply 1-2 drops to lower abdomen.

Application

Safety
Safe for neat application.

Key Properties
Tonic
Rubefacient
Neuroprotective
Calming
Carminative

Other Uses
Breast Enlargement, Depression, Irritability, Learning Difficulties, Memory Retention, Muscle Pain, Nerve Issues, Nervous Tension, PMS, Postpartum Depression, Restlessness, Termites, Workaholism

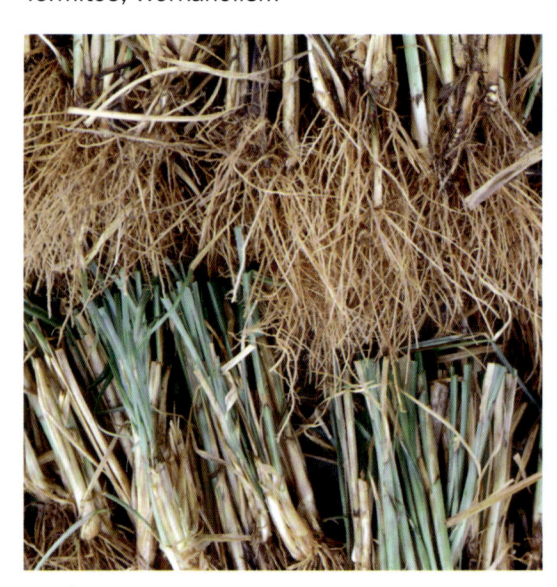

Wintergreen
Gaultheria Procumbens

Top Uses

Arthritis & Gout
Massage 1-2 drops neat or diluted into inflamed joints.

Muscle Pain & Inflammation
Massage 2-4 drops diluted into affected areas.

Broken Bones
Apply 1-2 drops gently over injury, avoiding open wounds.

Dandruff
Add a drop to shampoo, or massage 1-2 drops directly into scalp before shampooing.

Frozen Shoulder & Rotator Cuff
Massage 1-2 drops with carrier oil into affected area.

Teeth Whitening
Add a drop to a bit of baking soda, and brush twice daily until desired results are achieved.

Application

Safety
Dilute for sensitive skin.

Key Properties
Anti-inflammatory
Anti-rheumatic
Analgesic
Anti-spasmodic
Vasodilator

Other Uses
Bone Spurs, Cartilage Injury, Circulation, Muscle Development, Rheumatism

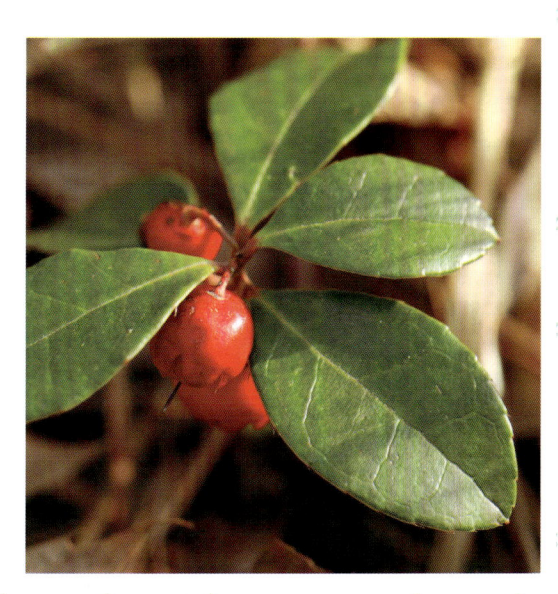

Ylang Ylang
Cananga Odorata

Top Uses

High Blood Pressure
Apply 2 drops to bottoms of feet, and take in a capsule daily.

Hormone Balance
Apply 1-2 drops to wrists and behind ears.

Low Libido
Apply 1-2 drops to pulse points and reproductive reflex points. Diffuse several drops during intimacy, or use in massage.

Oily Skin
Add a drop to toner or facial moisturizer, or take 1-2 drops in a capsule daily.

Infertility
Massage 1-2 drops over abdomen and reproductive reflex points.

Heart Palpitations
Rub 1-2 drops in a circular motion over heart. Also diffuse near bedside.

Application
A T I

Safety
Dilute for highly sensitive skin.

Key Properties
Hypotensive
Antispasmodic
Aphrodisiac
Sedative
Immunostimulant

Other Uses
Anxiety, Arterial Hypertension, Balance Issues, Chronic Fatigue, Circulation, Depression, Diabetes, Exhaustion, Hair Loss, Hypertension, Insomnia, Intestinal Spasms, Tachycardia

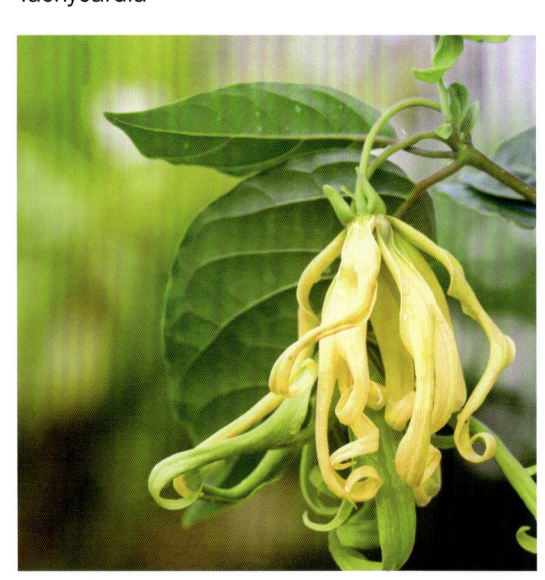

Oil Blends

Antioxidant Blend

Application

Top Uses

Free Radical Detox
Drink 1-3 drops in water or in a capsule, or apply to the bottoms of feet.

Chronic Cough
Rub 2-4 drops diluted over chest and mid-back. Also diffuse several drops.

Sore & Tense Muscles
Massage 2-4 drops diluted into affected muscles, being cautious of injuries.

Cognitive Performance
Inhale 1-2 drops from cupped hands, or diffuse several drops.

Cavities & Tooth Decay
Swish 2 drops with water as a mouthwash twice daily.

Immune Boost
Drink 1-3 drops in water or in a capsule, or apply to bottoms of feet.

Key Ingredients
Clove, Black Pepper, German Chamomile, Marjoram, Nutmeg

Other Uses
Cellulite, Colds, Creativity, Depression, Detox, Fear, Fluid Retention, Heart Palpitations, Insomnia, Menopause, Nervousness, Scurvy, Sluggish Digestion, Withdrawal Issues

Safety
Dilute for sensitive skin. Use with caution during pregnancy or if epileptic.

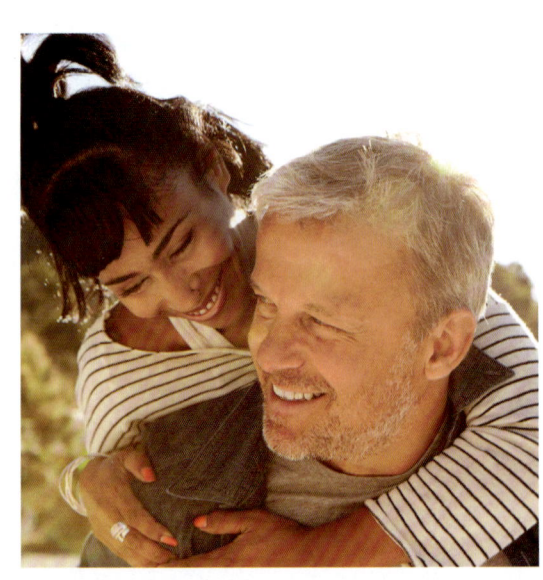

Oil Blends

Balancing Blend

Application

Top Uses

Stress
Rub 1-2 drops onto temples or pulse points.

Focus & Concentration
Apply 1-2 drops to the back of neck, or diffuse several drops.

Sleep Issues
Rub 1-2 drops to temples and bottoms of feet.

Skin Irritation
Apply a drop heavily diluted to irritated skin.

Epilepsy
Rub 1-2 drops onto the back of the neck and the bottoms of feet.

Irregular Menstruation
Massage a drop diluted over lower abdomen, and apply to bottoms of feet.

Key Ingredients
Mugwort, Cedarwood, Patchouli, Frankincense, Roman Chamomile, German Chamomile

Other Uses
Alzheimer's, Dementia, Diuretic, Hysteria, Meditation, Nervous System Conditions, Panic Attacks, Parkinson's, Seizures, Slow Digestion

Safety
Use caution during pregnancy and with infants.

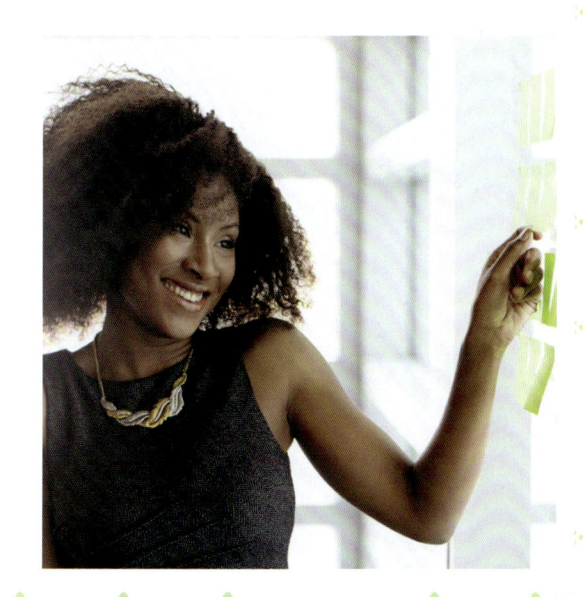

Oil Blends

Comforting Blend

Application A T I

Top Uses

Emotional Overwhelm
Inhale 1-2 drops from cupped hands, massage into back of neck, or diffuse.

Sleep Issues
Rub 1-2 drops into temples and bottoms of feet (focusing on big toes), and diffuse next to bedside.

Panic Attacks
Inhale 1-2 drops from cupped hands, and apply to temples.

Burns
Apply 1-2 drops diluted to burn areas, using extreme caution around damaged skin.

Nightmares
Diffuse 2-4 drops next to bedside.

Teething Pain
Massage a drop heavily diluted into baby's jawline, avoiding the mouth.

Key Ingredients
Lemon Verbena, Lavender, Bergamot, Ylang Ylang, Roman Chamomile, Sandalwood

Other Uses
Allergies, Anxiety, Burns, Depression, Hormone Balance, Irregular Menstruation, Menstrual Cramping, Muscle Spasms, Negative Thought Patterns, Swelling

Safety
Safe for neat application. Avoid UV exposure for 12 hours after topical application.

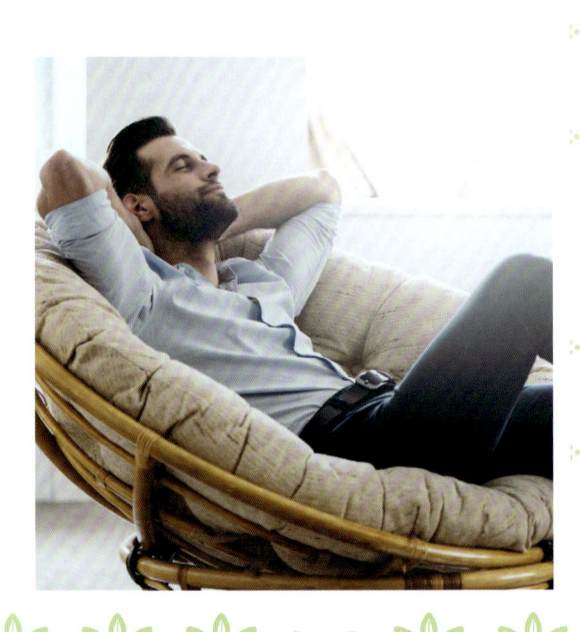

Concentration Blend

Application

Top Uses

Focus & Concentration
Apply 1-2 drops to temples and to the back of the neck.

Memory Retention
Diffuse several drops in the office or near a study space.

Nerve Support
Apply 2-4 drops to the bottoms of feet, focusing on the bony outside.

Cravings & Appetite
Diffuse several drops, or massage a drop into the stomach reflex point.

Bruises
Gently apply 1-2 drops to bruised area.

Key Ingredients
Wintergreen, Grapefruit, Vetiver

Other Uses
ADD/ADHD, Dizziness, Muscle Injury, Nervous Disorders

Safety
Dilute for sensitive skin. Use with caution during pregnancy.

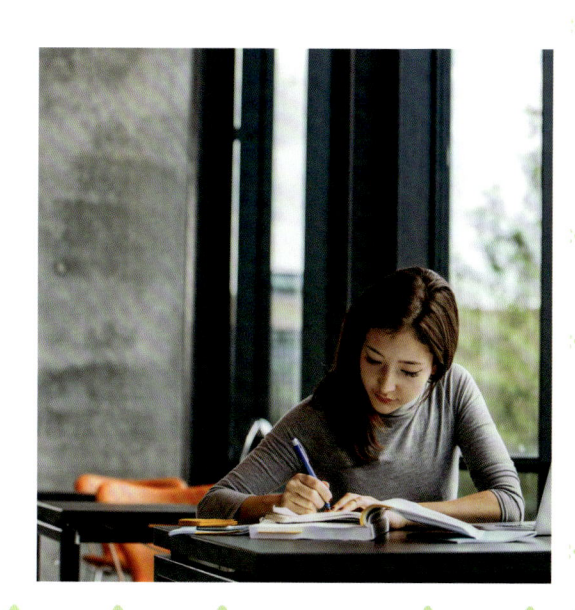

Oil Blends

Daily Cell Health Blend

Application

Top Uses

Cellular Vitality
Use internally in the morning and evening.

Mitochondria Performance
Use internally 3 times daily.

Cancer & Tumors
Use internally 5 times daily.

Autoimmune Disorders
Use internally 5 times daily.

Chronic Fatigue
Use internally 3 times daily.

Nutrient Utilization
Use internally in the morning and evening.

Key Ingredients
Lemongrass, Lavender, Ginger, Ylang Ylang, Balsam Fir, Clove, Oregano, Thyme, Black Pepper, German Chamomile, Marjoram, Nutmeg, Helichrysum

Other Uses
Antioxidant, Immune Boost

Safety
Use with caution when taking with several medications.

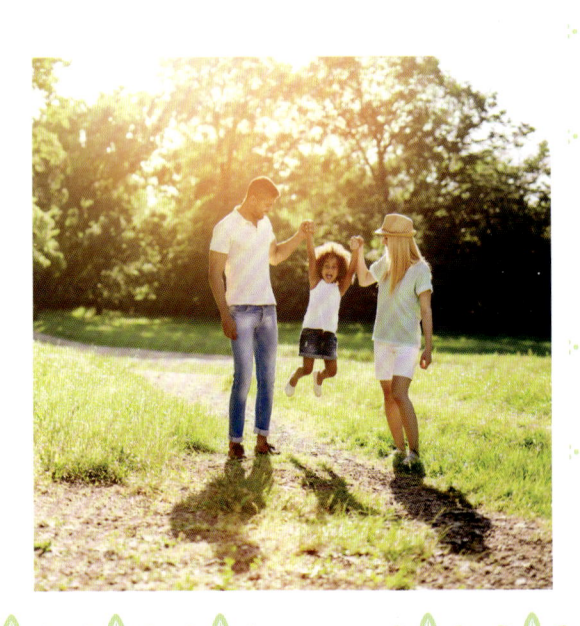

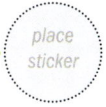

Daily Digestive Blend

Application

Top Uses

Sluggish Digestion
Use internally with each meal.

Stomach Upset
Use internally at the onset of an upset stomach.

Intestinal Spasms
Use a double dose internally at the onset of uncomfortable spasms.

Intestinal Parasites
Use internally 5 times daily.

Irregular Bowel Movements
Use internally with each meal.

Key Ingredients
Spruce, Peppermint, Orange, Thyme, Marjoram, Lemon, Vetiver

Other Uses
ADD/ADHD, Anxiety, Depression, Mood swings

Safety
Use caution while breastfeeding or if epileptic.

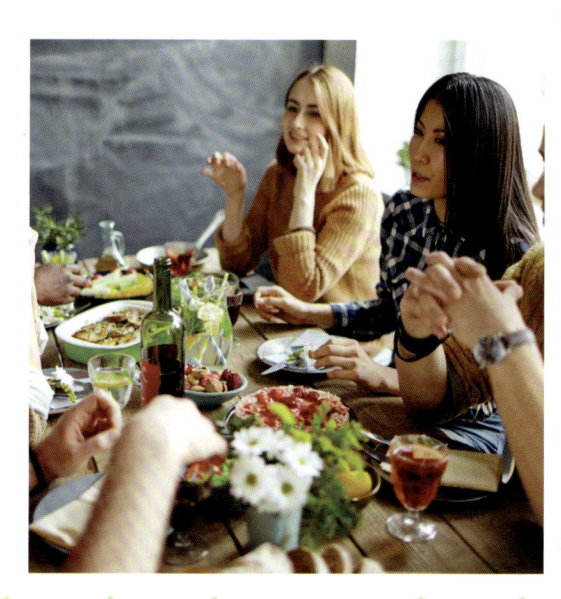

Oil Blends

Detoxification Blend

Application A T I

Top Uses

Endocrine System Support
Drink 2-4 drops in water or a capsule morning and evening.

Immunostimulant
Drink 1-2 drops in water, or apply to the bottoms of feet.

Liver & Kidney Detox
Drink 1-3 drops in water, and rub over the liver and kidneys.

Candida
Drink 1-3 drops in water 3 times daily, and rub on bottoms of feet.

Sugar Toxicity
Drink 1-3 drops in water, and rub on bottoms of feet and over pancreas.

Key Ingredients
Lavender, Frankincense, Eucalyptus

Other Uses
Alzheimer's, Bacterial Infection, Burns, Cough, Diabetes (type 2), Focus Issues, Hyperthyroidism, Viral Infection

Safety
Safe for neat application. Avoid use with infants.

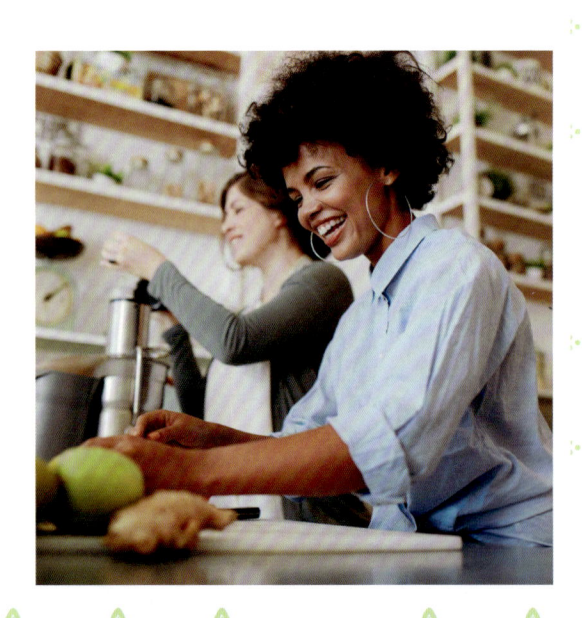

Digestive Support Blend

Application

Top Uses

Upset Stomach
Drink 1-3 drops in water, or rub over stomach in a clockwise motion.

Gas & Flatulence
Drink 1-3 drops in water or in a capsule.

Constipation
Drink 1-3 drops in water, and rub over outside of stomach and on stomach reflex points.

Diarrhea
Drink 1-3 drops in water or in a capsule.

Diverticulitis
Drink 1-3 drops in water, and rub over outside of stomach and lower abdomen.

Crohn's Disease
Drink 1-3 drops in water to help manage pain if a flareup occurs.

Key Ingredients
Ginger, Peppermint, Orange, Spruce, Thyme, Fennel, Marjoram, Lemon, Vetiver

Other Uses
Cold, Cough, Flu, Nausea, Morning Sickness, Motion Sickness, Parasites, Vomiting

Safety
Use caution during pregnancy and breast feeding.

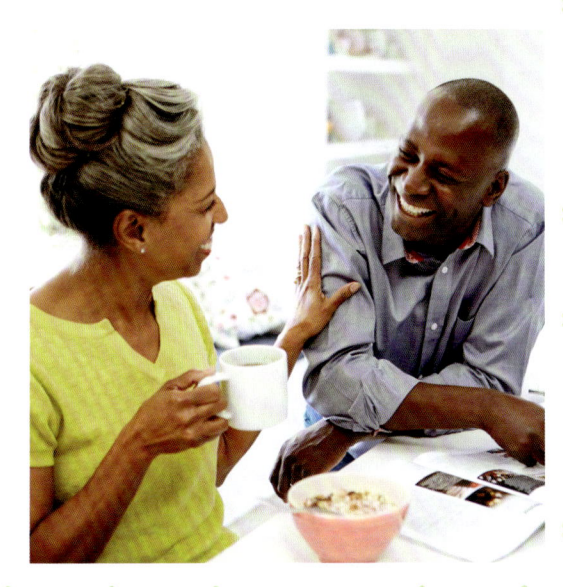

Oil Blends

Focusing Blend

Application A T I

Top Uses

Focus & Concentration
Rub 1-2 drops onto temples and back of neck.

Grounding & Meditation
Rub 1-2 drops behind ears and onto bottoms of feet.

Energetic/Emotional Toxicity
Diffuse several drops, and rub 1-3 drops over heart and sacrum.

Ear Infection
Place a drop on a cotton ball, and rest over ear for 15 minutes. Also apply behind ear.

ADD/ADHD
Apply 1-3 drops to back of neck, rub onto bottoms of feet, or diffuse several drops.

Vitality & Well-Being
Inhale 1-2 drops from cupped hands, or diffuse several drops.

Key Ingredients
Sandalwood, Rosewood, Sage, Juniper Berry, Spearmint

Other Uses
Bladder Infection, Dermatitis, Eczema, Hyperactivity, Learning Disorders, Psoriasis, Scar Tissue, Urinary Infection, Vaginal Infection

Safety
Safe for neat application.

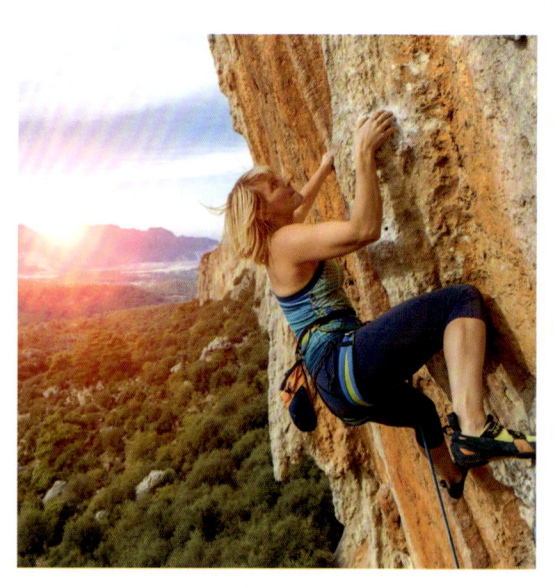

Immunity-Boosting Blend

Application

Top Uses

Cold & Flu
Drink 1-3 drops in water, and apply to bottoms of feet.

Intestinal Parasites
Drink 2-4 drops in water or a capsule 3-5 times daily for 5 days.

Sore Throat
Gargle 2 drops with water.

Candida
Drink 1-3 drops in water or in a capsule 3-5 times daily for 7 days.

Bacterial Infections
Drink 1-3 drops in water or in a capsule.

Food Poisoning
Drink 1-3 drops in water or in a capsule every 30 minutes until symptoms subside, up to 3 hours.

Key Ingredients
Oregano, Thyme, Lemongrass, Ginger, Helichrysum, Ylang Ylang

Other Uses
Airborne Pathogens, Antioxidant, Control Issues, Diverticulitis, Fungal Infections, Lactose Intolerance, Mold, MRSA, Serotonin Depletion, Stomach Ulcers, Tonsillitis, Viral Infections

Safety
Dilute for topical use. Use with caution if pregnant or epileptic.

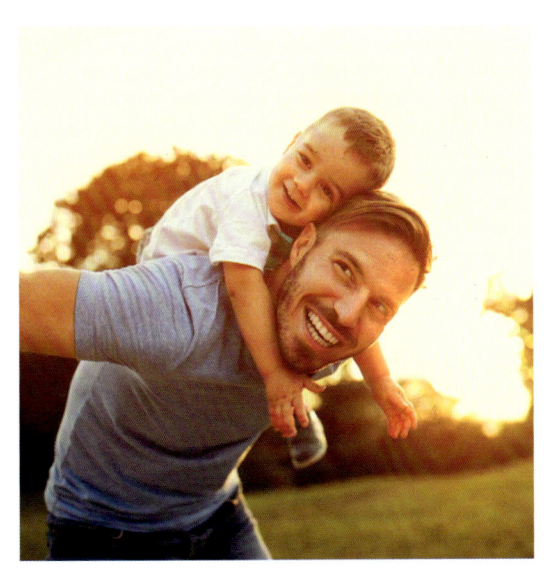

Oil Blends

Massage Blend

Application

Top Uses

Muscle Tension
Massage 2-4 drops with carrier oil into affected muscles.

Headache & Migraine
Rub 1-2 drops into temples and base of skull.

Back, Neck, & Shoulder Pain
Massage 2-4 drops into sore muscles.

Arthritis & Joint Pain
Massage 1-3 drops into painful joints.

Connective Tissue Damage
Carefully massage 2-4 drops into damaged ligaments & tendons.

Circulation Issues
Rub 1-2 drops onto bottoms of feet.

High Blood Pressure
Rub 1-2 drops onto bottoms of feet, and diffuse several drops.

Key Ingredients
Lavender, Black Pepper, Peppermint, Wintergreen, Basil, Roman Chamomile, Eucalyptus, Rosemary

Other Uses
Cold Extremities, Cough, Cramping, Lymphatic Support, Neuropathy, Restless Leg Syndrome

Safety
Dilute for sensitive skin. Use with caution during pregnancy and breast feeding.

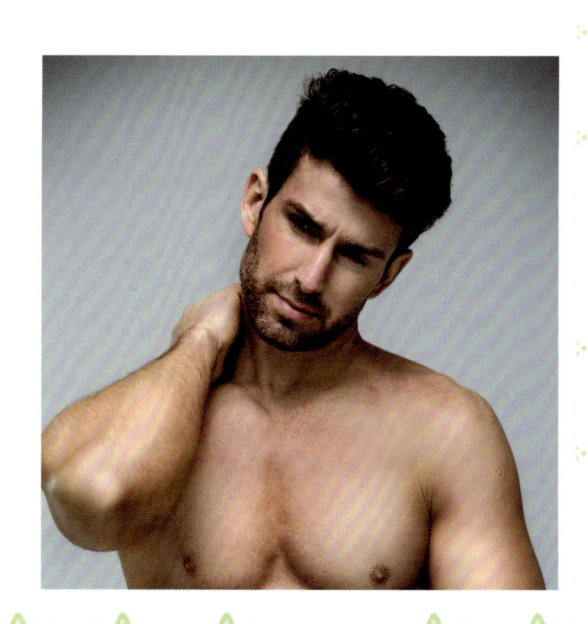

Men's Daily Balancing Blend

Application

Top Uses

Male Hormone Balance
Use internally morning and evening.

Low Testosterone
Use internally morning and evening, and 30 minutes before exercise.

Adrenal Fatigue
Use internally morning and evening.

Premature Aging
Use internally morning and evening.

Key Ingredients
Basil, Tea Tree, Bergamot, Clove, Eucalyptus, Vetiver

Other Uses
Food Poisoning, Immune Support, Intestinal Infections, Intestinal Spasms, Irritability

Safety
Safe for internal use.

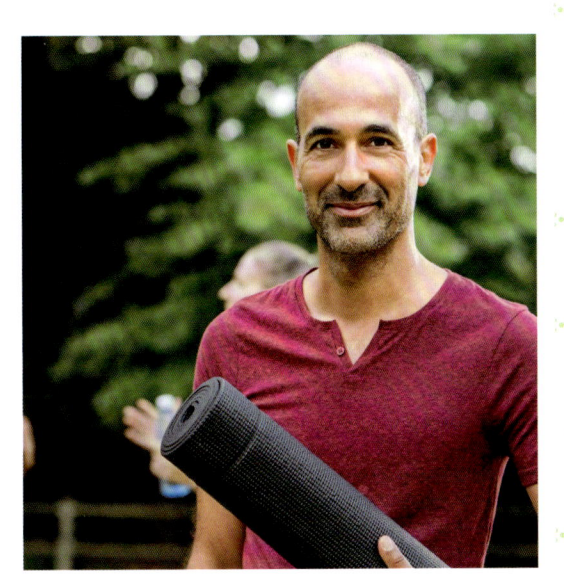

Monthly Blend

Application

Top Uses

PMS
Apply 1-2 drops to wrists and lower abdomen.

Menstrual Cramping
Massage 1-3 drops over lower abdomen.

Mood Swings
Apply 1-2 drops to pulse points, and diffuse several drops.

Excessive Menstruation
Apply 2-4 drops to bottoms of feet, and also rub over abdomen.

Menopause
Apply 1-2 drops to pulse points.

Low Sex Drive
Apply 1-2 drops to pulse points, and diffuse several drops during intimacy.

Key Ingredients
Clary Sage, Bergamot, Rosemary, Lavender, Frankincense, Fennel, Nutmeg, Clove, Lemon, Ylang Ylang, Tea Tree

Other Uses
Hormone Irregularities, Hot Flashes, Pre-Menopause, Rashes, Skin Conditions

Safety
Avoid UV exposure for 12 hours after topical application. Use with caution during pregnancy.

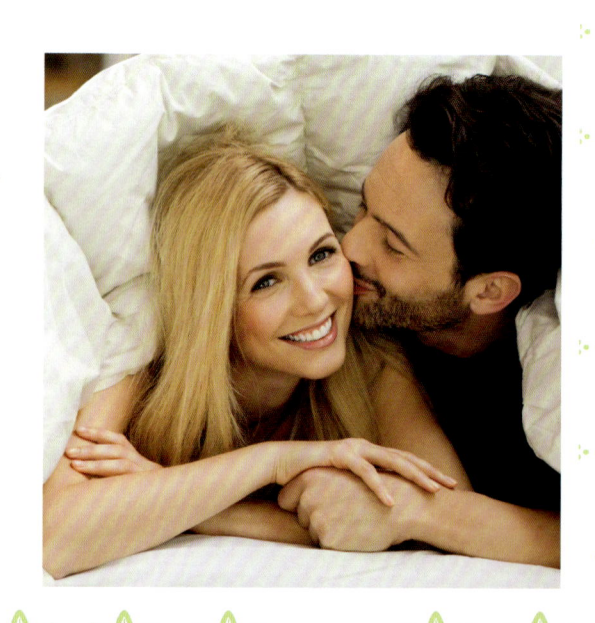

Nourishing Blend

Application

Top Uses

Cancer & Tumors
Drink 1-3 drops in water, or apply diluted to the affected area often.

Damaged DNA
Drink 1-3 drops in water, or apply to bottoms of feet.

Estrogen & Progesterone Issues
Apply 1-2 drops to bottoms of feet in the morning and evening.

Seizures
Apply 1-3 drops to the bottoms of feet.

Nerve Damage
Massage 1-3 drops into the bottoms of feet and along spine.

Autoimmune Disorders
Apply 1-3 drops to the bottoms of feet and along spine, and drink in water or in a capsule.

Key Ingredients
Lemongrass, Lavender, Ginger, Ylang Ylang, Balsam Fir

Other Uses
Brain Degradation, Candida, Detox, Fungal Hypothyroidism, Infections, Inflammation, Viral Infections

Safety
Dilute for topical use. Use with caution during pregnancy or if epileptic.

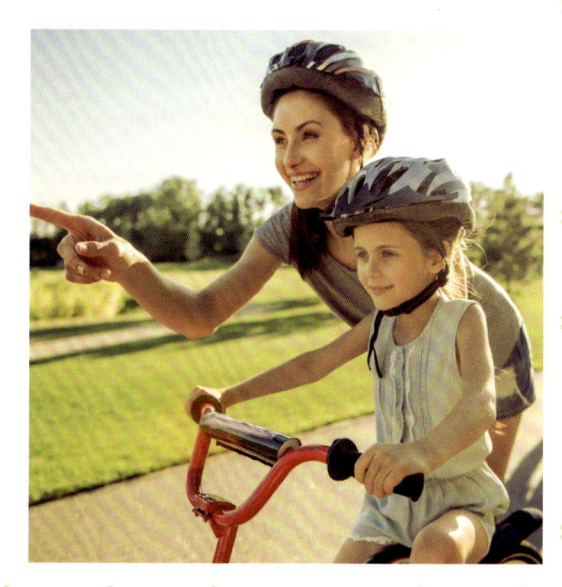

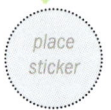

Protecting Blend

Application A T I

Top Uses

Cold & Flu
Drink 1-3 drops in water or in a capsule, and rub onto the bottoms of feet.

Bacterial & Viral Infections
Drink 1-3 drops in water or in a capsule.

Airborne Pathogens
Diffuse several drops.

Strep Throat & Tonsillitis
Gargle 2 drops with water for 30 seconds, then swallow.

Cold Sores
Apply a drop diluted to affected areas.

Parasite Issues
Drink 1-3 drops in water or in a capsule 3-5 times a day for 7 days.

Key Ingredients
Clove, Cinnamon, Lemongrass, Orange, Lemon, Rosemary, Eucalyptus

Other Uses
Air Purification, Autoimmune Disorders, Chronic Fatigue, Cough, Gum Disease, Mildew, Mold, Urinary Infection

Safety
Dilute for sensitive skin.

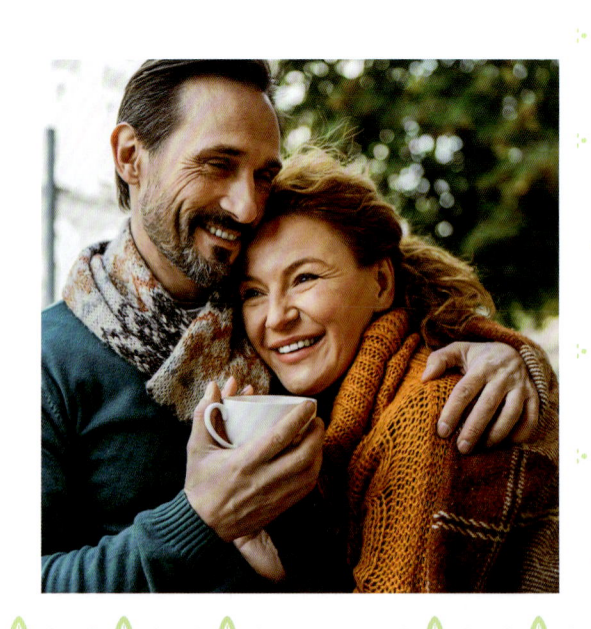

Purifying Blend

Application

Top Uses

Air Purification
Diffuse several drops.

Laundry Freshener
Add 3-6 drops to washing machine.

Mold & Mildew
Add several drops to a glass spray bottle with water, and apply before scrubbing.

Insect Repellent
Apply diluted to exposed skin during outdoor activities.

Household Cleaner
Add several drops to distilled water in a glass spray bottle to disinfect surfaces.

Halitosis
Add a drop to your toothbrush to kill germs in the mouth.

Key Ingredients
Orange, Lemon, Citronella, Vanilla, Thyme, Lime

Other Uses
Bug Bites, Cuts, Mental Fatigue, Mildew in Air Filters, Pimples, Scrapes,

Safety
Avoid UV exposure for 12 hours after topical application.

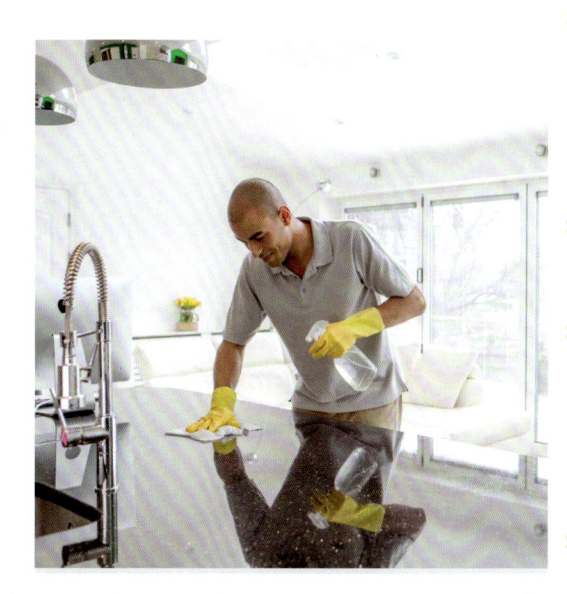

Oil Blends

Respiration Blend

Application

Top Uses

Asthma
Inhale 1-3 drops from cupped hands, and apply to lung reflex points.

Allergies
Inhale 1-2 drops from cupped hands, or diffuse several drops.

Bronchitis & Pneumonia
Rub 2-4 drops diluted to chest and mid-back, and diffuse several drops.

Snoring
Apply a drop over throat and sinuses, avoiding the eyes. Also diffuse next to bedside.

Cough
Inhale 1-2 drops from cupped hands, and apply to chest.

Cardio & Exercise
Apply 2-4 drops to chest before exercising.

Key Ingredients
Balsam Fir, Eucalyptus, Marjoram, Sandalwood, Myrtle, Oregano

Other Uses
Altitude Change, Exercise-Induced Asthma, Mucus, Phlegm

Safety
Dilute for sensitive skin. Use caution if pregnant. Avoid topical use with infants.

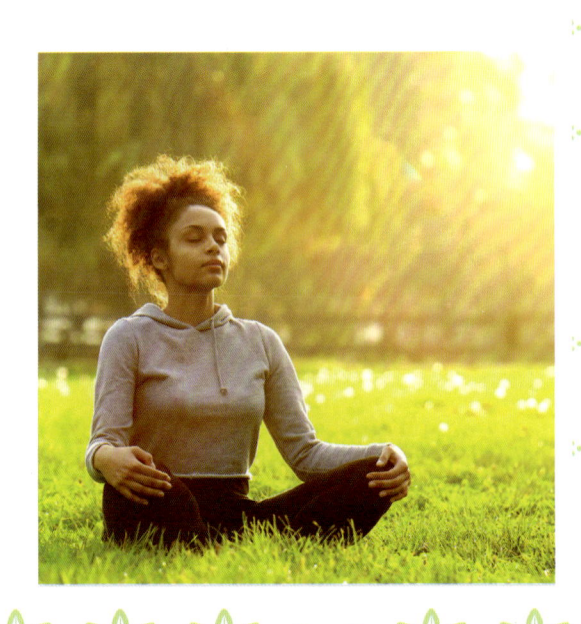

Respiratory Blend

Application

Top Uses

Cough
Inhale 1-3 drops from cupped hands, and rub over chest.

Congestion
Rub 2-4 drops over chest and mid-back.

Panic Attacks
Deeply and slowly inhale 1-2 drops from cupped hands.

Mental Clarity
Inhale 1-2 drops from cupped hands, and diffuse several drops.

Circulation Issues
Apply 1-3 drops to bottoms of feet morning and evening.

Fever
Apply 1-2 drops to back of neck and shoulders.

Key Properties
Eucalyptus Globulus, Eucalyptus Radiata, Ravintsara, Rosemary, Frankincense, Cypress, Peppermint, Cajeput

Other Uses
Asthma, Chronic Cough, Exercise Induced Asthma, Jet Lag, Mucus, Pneumonia, Shortness of Breath, Weak Lungs

Safety
Dilute for use on sensitive skin. Use caution if pregnant. Avoid topical use on infants.

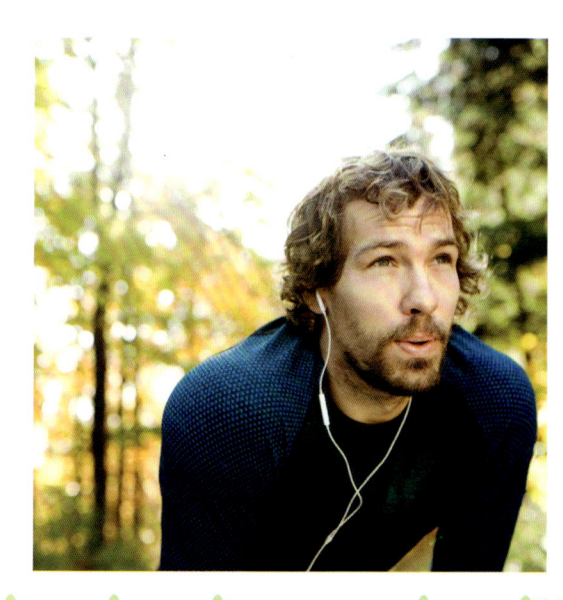

Oil Blends

131

Restorative Blend

Application

Top Uses

Bruises
Apply 1-2 drops to bruised skin several times throughout the day.

Muscle Aches & Fatigue
Massage 2-4 drops diluted into affected muscles.

Cuts & Scrapes
Apply a drop diluted to affected skin every few hours.

Fatigue
Rub 1-3 drops over adrenals, sides of throat, and temples.

Meditation Enhancement
Apply 1-2 drops to wrists and pulse points during meditation.

Chronic Pain
Apply 1-3 drops to bottoms of feet and pulse points, and diffuse several drops.

Key Ingredients
Copaiba, Spruce, Cedarwood, Frankincense, Rosemary, Lavender, Geranium, German Chamomile

Other Uses
ADD, Charley Horse, Congestion, Emotional Toxicity, Exercise Recovery, Focus, Muscle Injury, PTSD, Scarring, Stress

Safety
Safe for neat application

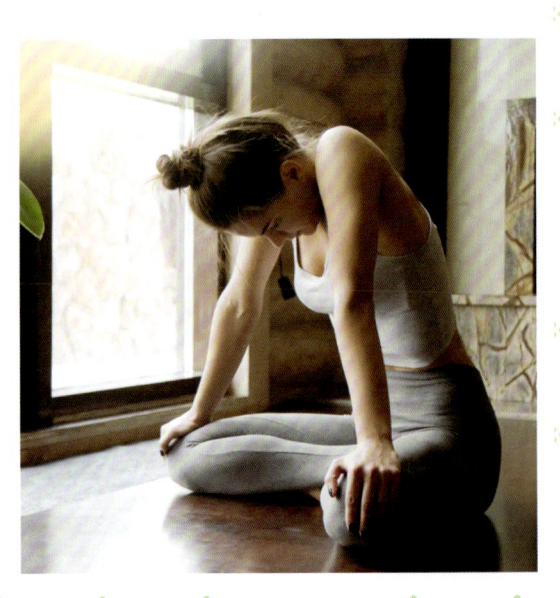

Skin-Enriching Blend

Application

Top Uses

Scar Tissue
Massage 1-2 drops into scar tissue morning and at bedtime.

Psoriasis
Apply 1-2 drops diluted to affected areas, and apply to bottoms of feet daily.

Wrinkles & Fine Lines
Add 1-2 drops to daily facial moisturizer.

Large Pores
Add a drop to facial toner.

Loss of Skin Elasticity
Add 1-2 drops to carrier oil or regular coconut oil, and massage into loose skin.

Hormone Imbalance
Apply 1-2 drops to pulse points.

Anxiety
Rub 1-2 drops into temples and wrists, or diffuse several drops.

Key Ingredients
Ylang Ylang, Bergamot, Cypress, Rosemary, Helichrysum

Other Uses
Aphrodisiac, Cuts & Scrapes, Emotional Fatigue, Mental Fog, Stress-Related Conditions

Safety
Avoid direct UV exposure 12 hours after topical use.

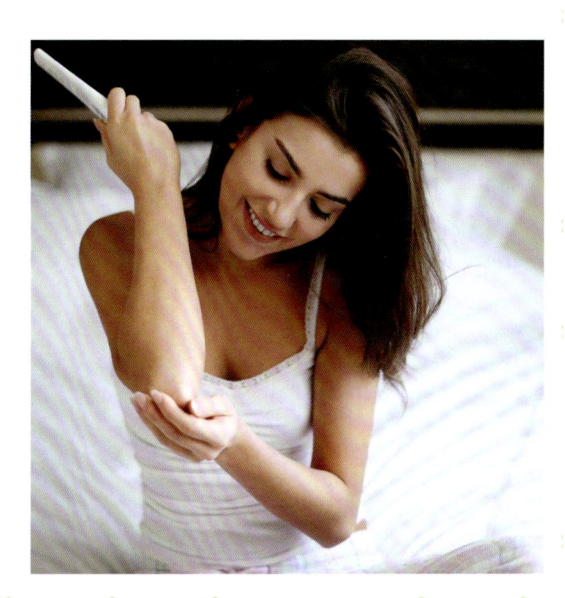

Oil Blends

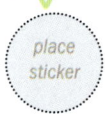

Slimming Blend

Application

Top Uses

Cravings
Add 4-8 drops to water and drink throughout the day. Also diffuse several drops.

Cellulite
Add 12-20 drops to a carrier oil and massage into areas with cellulite. Wait 20 minutes before showering. Repeat frequently.

Toxicity
Drink 1-3 drops in water, and apply to bottoms of feet.

Lethargy
Drink 4-8 drops in water throughout the day, or diffuse several drops.

Metabolism Boost
Drink 4-8 drops in water throughout the day, especially before exercise.

Addiction
Drink 4-8 drops in water throughout the day, and apply to bottoms of feet.

Key Ingredients
Orange, Tangerine, Lemon, Black Pepper, Spearmint, Grapefruit, Peppermint

Other Uses
Chronic Fatigue, Depression, Diabetes, Energy, Self-Consciousness, Viruses

Safety
Avoid direct UV exposure for 12 hours after topical application.

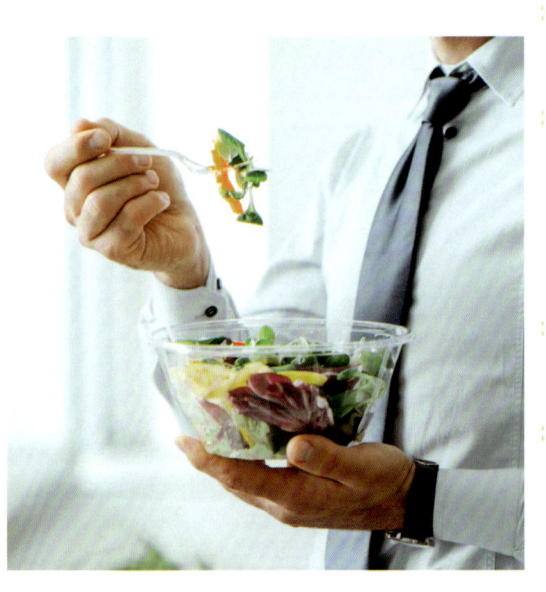

Soothing Blend

Application

Top Uses

Back, Neck, & Shoulder Pain
Massage 2-4 drops diluted into painful muscle areas.

Arthritis & Joint Pain
Massage 1-3 drops into affected areas.

Lupus & Fibromyalgia
Apply 2-4 drops diluted over painful areas during a flareup.

Tension Headache
Massage 1-2 drops into temples (avoiding the eyes) and the back of neck.

Muscle Aches
Massage 2-4 drops diluted into affected muscles.

Muscle Injury
Apply 1-3 drops over affected muscles, avoiding too much pressure.

Key Ingredients
Wintergreen, Spruce, Peppermint, Helichrysum Camphor, Balsam Fir

Other Uses
Asthma, Brain Fog, Bronchitis, Bruising, Circulation, Cough, Hot Flashes, Gout, Inflammation, Rheumatism, Tendinitis

Safety
Dilute for sensitive skin. Use with caution during pregnancy and breast feeding.

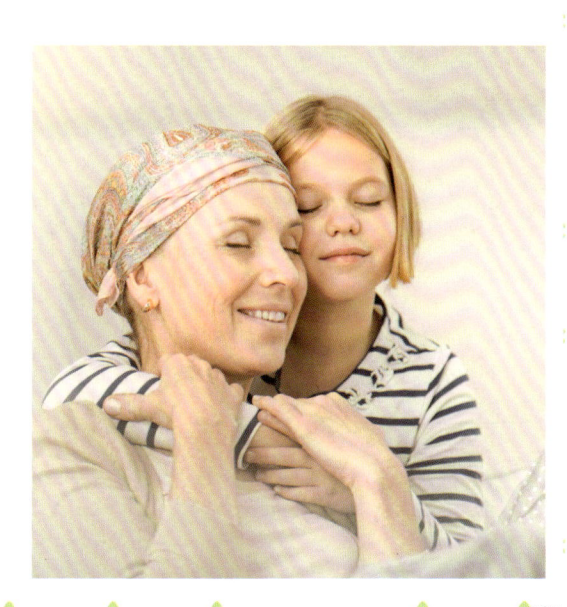

Stress Control Blend

Application

Top Uses

Anxiety
Inhale 1-2 drops from cupped hands, and wear on pulse points.

ADD/ADHD
Rub 1-2 drops onto back of neck and temples.

Hyperactivity
Diffuse several drops, or apply 1-3 drops to the bottoms of feet.

Sleep Issues
Rub 1-2 drops onto temples and bottoms of feet, rub a drop over pillow, or diffuse a few drops by bedside.

Emotional Overwhelm
Inhale 1-2 drops from cupped hands, and rub over heart.

Neck & Shoulder Pain
Massage 2-4 drops diluted into neck and shoulders.

Key Ingredients
Copaiba Balsam, Cedarwood, Pine, Neroli, Lavandin, Lime, Lavender, Lemon Verbena

Other Uses
Cradle Cap, Depression, Dysphagia, Fear, Fluid Retention, Heart Palpitations, Insomnia, Menopause, Nervousness, Sluggish Digestion, Withdrawal Issues

Safety
Safe for neat application.

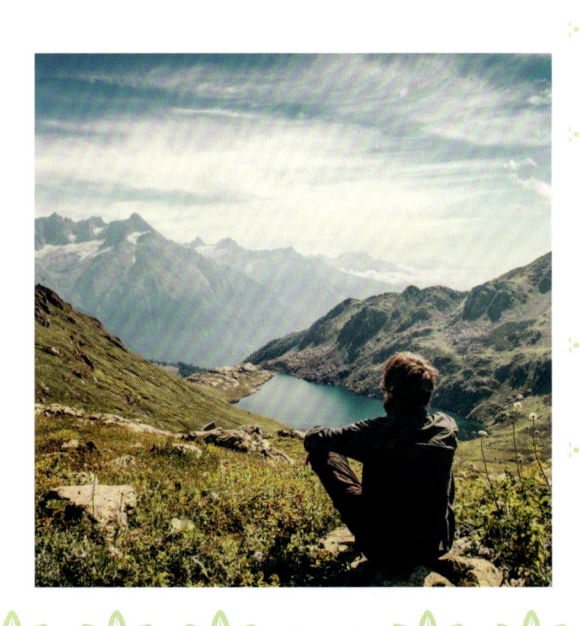

Vitality-Boosting Blend

Application

Top Uses

Energy
Drink 1-3 drops in water, or inhale from cupped hands.

Depression
Inhale 1-2 drops from cupped hands, or diffuse several drops.

Hypothyroidism
Apply 1-2 drops over thyroid, diluting for sensitive skin.

Antioxidant
Drink 1-3 drops in water, or apply to bottoms of feet.

Intestinal Parasites
Drink 3-6 drops in water or a capsule 3-5 times daily for 7 days.

Viruses
Drink 1-3 drops in water, apply to bottoms of feet, or diffuse several drops.

Key Ingredients
Tangerine, Orange, Clove

Other Uses
Colds, Flu, Herpes, Hodgkin's Disease, Jaundice, Lipoma, Lyme Disease, Smoking Addiction, Stress-Induced Issues, Water Retention, Weight Loss

Safety
Avoid UV exposure for 12 hours after topical application.

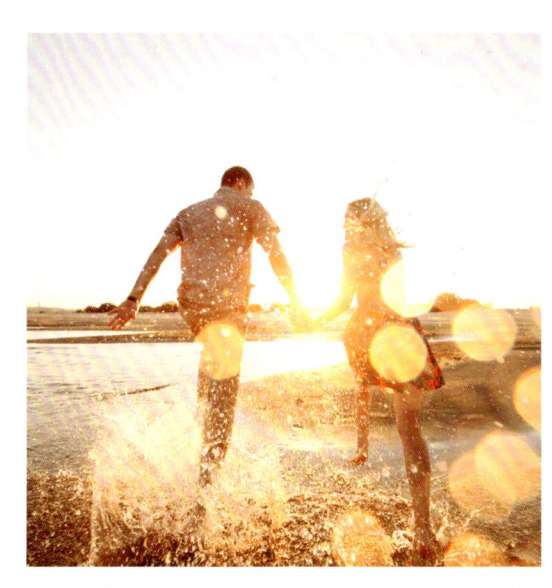

Oil Blends

Weight Control Blend

Application

Top Uses

Metabolism Boost
Drink 2-4 drops in water, and rub 1-2 drops over pancreas and bottoms of feet.

Energy
Inhale 1-2 drops from cupped hands, or diffuse several drops.

Craving Control
Drink 2-4 drops in water throughout the day, or place a drop under the tongue.

Adrenal Fatigue
Rub 1-2 drops neat over adrenals.

Stomach Upset
Drink 1-3 drops in water, or rub over stomach in a clockwise motion.

Eating Disorders
Inhale 1-2 drops from cupped hands, drink 2-4 drops in water, and diffuse several drops.

Key Ingredients
Lemon, Roman Chamomile, Basil, Ginger

Other Uses
Congestion, Chronic Cough, Chronic Fatigue, Constipation, Detoxification, Digestive Disorders, Heart Palpitations, Immune System Boost, Mood Disorders, Phlegm

Safety
Avoid UV exposure for 12 hours after topical application. Dilute for sensitive skin.

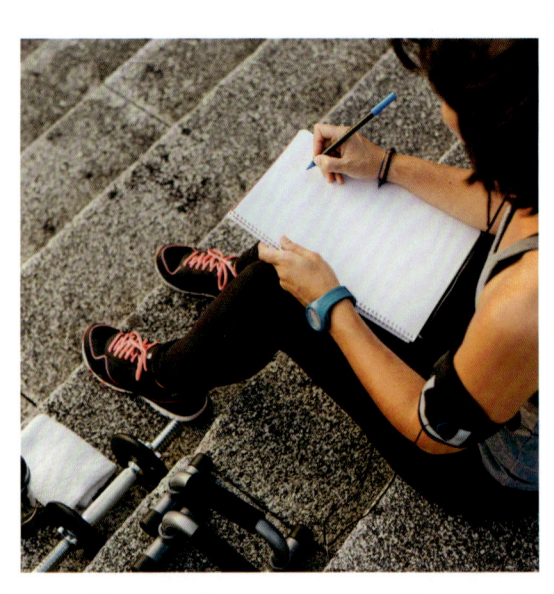

Women's Daily Balancing Blend

Application

Top Uses

Hormone Balance
Use internally morning and evening.

Infertility
Use internally 3-5 times daily.

PMS & Menopause
Use internally with each meal.

Irritable Bowel Syndrome
Use internally 20 minutes before eating.

Candida
Use internally 3-5 times daily for 10 days, then return to morning and evening use.

Key Ingredients
Rosemary, Lemon, Vetiver, Bergamot, Clove, Tea Tree

Other Uses
Alzheimer's, Bacterial Infections, Diuretic, Heart Issues, Intestinal Pain, Mucus, Multiple Sclerosis, Parasites, Nervous Disorders, Vaginal Infection

Safety
Use with caution during pregnancy.

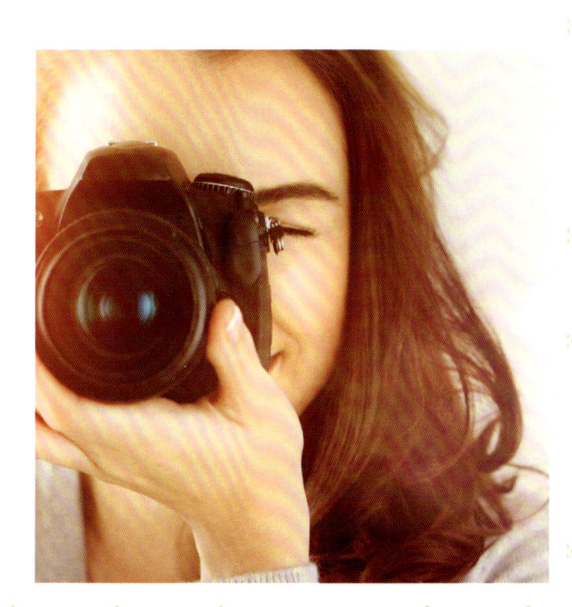

Protocols

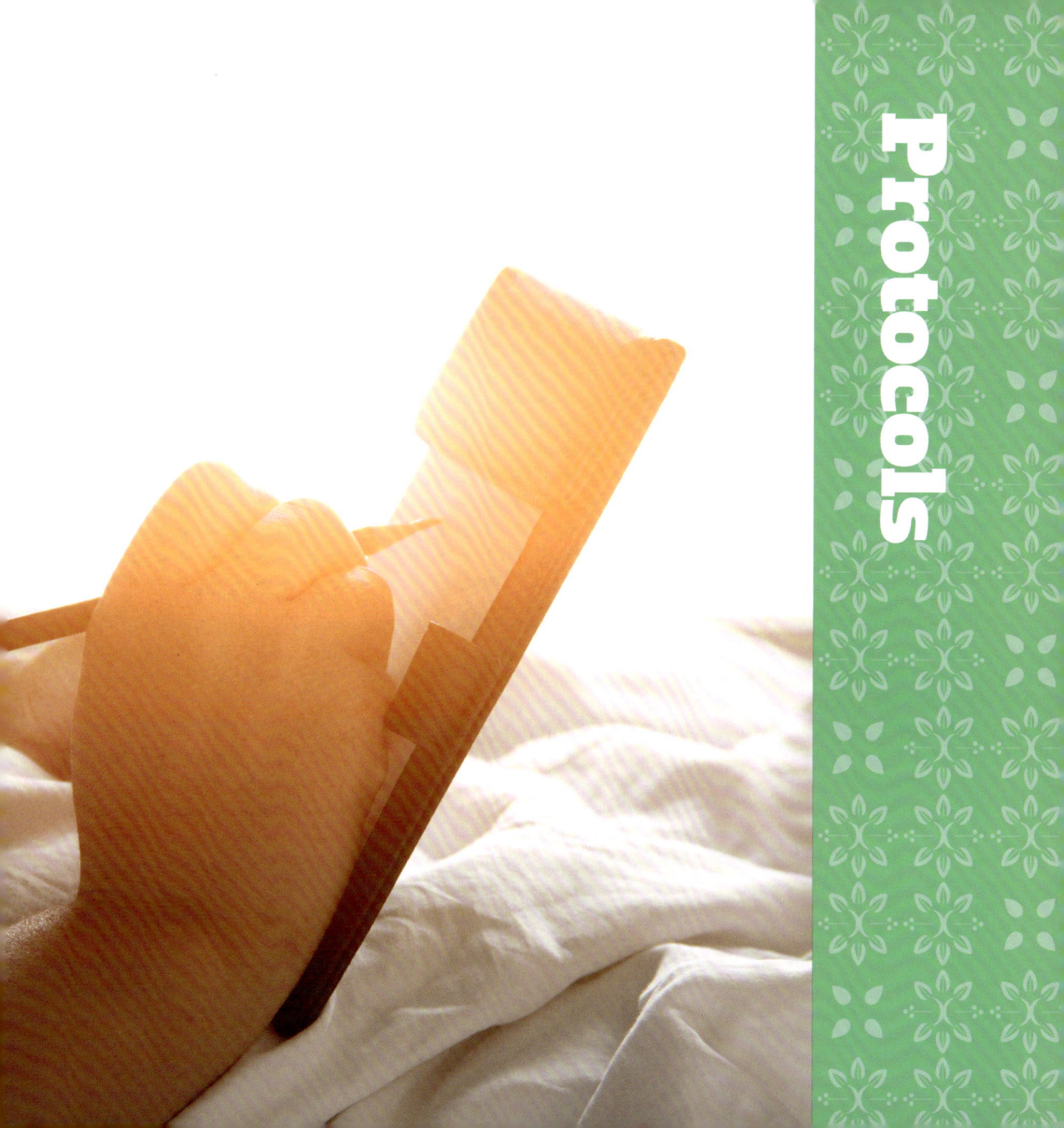

Acne (bacteria)

Combats bacterial issues that become trapped in pores.

Suggested Duration
Ongoing

Skin-Enriching Blend
Apply a small amount evenly over clean skin after showering daily.

Tea Tree
Apply a dab to blemishes.

Frankincense
Apply a dab to heal blemishes, and to prevent scarring.

Also Try
- Helichrysum

Acne (hormonal)

Balances hormone production and maintenance throughout the body, including the gut.

Suggested Duration
Until desired appearance is achieved, then as needed.

Moringa Super Powder
Use one pouch of mix daily as directed.

Clary Sage
Rub 1 drop onto pulse points before bed.

Monthly Blend
Apply 2 drops to bottoms of feet morning and night (for men and women)

Tea Tree
Apply a dab to blemishes.

Also Try
- Ylang Ylang

Acne (toxicity)

Stimulates thyroid in order to produce proper hormones.

Suggested Duration
3-5 weeks

Premium Tea
Use tea nightly 30 minutes before bed. Try adding a drop of lemon oil to tea.

Detoxification Blend
Rub 2-4 drops on bottoms of feet before showering in mornings, as well as before bed.

Antioxidant Blend
Rub 2 drops over liver and kidneys, and drink 2 drops in water or a capsule twice daily.

Also Try
A 30-day full body detox is highly recommended, including eliminating sugars and dairy.

ADD/ADHD

Increases focus and concentration, supports healthy hormones and brain chemistry.

Suggested Duration
Ongoing

Nitric Oxide Activator
Use activator daily as directed to stimulate healthy neurological function.

Moringa Super Powder
Use Moringa daily to supply the brain needed nutrients.

Vetiver
Apply a dab behind ears as needed.

Frankincense
Apply a drop to the roof of the mouth in the morning.

Restorative Blend
Inhale 1-2 drops from cupped hands often to increase focus.

Adrenal Fatigue

Supports healthy adrenal function.

Suggested Duration
4-8 weeks

Extreme Moringa Energy
Use Moringa energy daily as directed.

Limitless Energy Powder
Use energy mix for an emergency pick-me-up.

Lemon (8 drops), Basil (3), Rosemary (3), Frankincense (3)
Combine in roller bottle. Fill the rest with carrier oil. Massage into neck and over adrenals daily as often as needed.

Rosemary & Peppermint
Breathe a drop of each from cupped hands, or diffuse for energy as needed.

AIDS/HIV

Provides emotional support, promotes a properly functioning immune system.

Suggested Duration
6 months, then as needed

Moringa Super Powder
Use Moringa daily as directed.

Vitality-Boosting Blend
Carry with you, and inhale from cupped hands for daily emotional support.

Nourishing Blend
Rub 3-5 drops into spine nightly.

Antioxidant Blend
Take 3-5 drops in a capsule daily.

Protecting Blend
Rub 2 drops on bottoms of feet daily to combat threats.

Also Try
- Oregano & Frankincense

Allergies (food)

Lowers histamine response triggered by food allergies; creates calm in the gut.

Suggested Duration
4 weeks to begin, then as needed

Lavender
Put 1 drop under tongue. Drink water after 30 seconds.

Premium Tea
Use daily to eliminate toxins from the gut.

Helichrysum
Take 2-4 drops in a capsule twice daily to help heal leaky gut.

Also Try
- Bone broth protein from the health food store
- Frankincense

Allergies (pet/seasonal)

Reduces histamine response and boosts immune system.

Suggested Duration
4-8 weeks to begin, then as needed

Extreme Moringa Energy
Use daily to enhance immune system.

Lemon, Lavender, Peppermint
Put 1 drop of each under the tongue during flare-ups. Drink water after 30 seconds.

Respiratory Blend
Inhale 1-3 from cupped hands, and rub carefully over bridge of nose.

Protecting Blend
Gargle 2 drops with water nightly, then swallow.

Also Try
- Scotch Pine
- Respiration Bend

Alzheimer's & Dementia

Supports healthy mental activity; boosts alertness.

Suggested Duration
Ongoing

Nitric Oxide Activator
Use daily to boost mental alertness and cognitive function.

Moringa Super Powder
Use daily to provide plant-based nutrients to the brain.

Nourishing Blend
Rub 4 drops along spine nightly.

Peppermint & Rosemary
Diffuse a few drops of each to increase alertness and memory.

Also Try
- Frankincense
- Balancing Blend

Anxiety

Reduces stress levels; promotes a sense of calm, security, and focus.

Suggested Duration
3-6 months, then as needed

Premium Tea
Use tea nightly to ease stress from the day.

Stress Control Blend
Apply a coupe drops to pulse points and inhale from cupped hands as needed throughout the day.

Balancing Blend
Apply 2 drops to the bottoms of feet each morning to start the day grounded.

Also Try
- Comforting Blend
- Patchouli
- Lavender
- Orange

Arthritis

Reduces inflammation in joints; supports joint function.

Suggested Duration
8 weeks to start, then as needed

Optimal Aging Blend
Use daily to manage inflammation.

Moringa Super Powder
Use daily to provide needed omegas for healthy joints.

Soothing Blend
Massage 2 drops into painful joints as often as needed.

Nourishing Blend
Massage 2 drops into problematic joints each morning.

Also Try
- Lemongrass
- Massage Blend
- Wintergreen
- Restorative Blend

Asthma

Promotes open airways and easy breathing; calms stress of asthmatic attack.

Suggested Duration
As needed

Nitric Oxide Activator
Use daily to promote healthy cardiovascular function.

Respiration Blend
Rub 2-4 drops along spine and bottoms of feet to encourage healthy gene expression for respiratory health. Also inhale 2 drops from cupped hands during attacks.

Lavender
Massage 1-2 drops behind ears to promote calm.

Also Try
- Rosemary
- Spearmint
- Balsam Fir

Protocols

Athletic Support

Provides natural stimulants and nutrients to support exercise and building lean muscle mass.

Suggested Duration
Ongoing, especially during exercise sprees

Extreme Moringa Energy
Use daily to provide needed nutrients and energy factors.

Nitric Oxide Activator
Use daily to support body system function and cardiovascular heath.

Plant Protein
Use after each workout, or as a supplement/replacement for breakfast.

AM/PM Caps
Use to support exercise and healthy appetite.

Vitality-Boosting Blend
Rub 2 drops onto pulse points for a sense of vitality.

Autism

Promotes high-functioning mental activity; reduces heavy metal toxicity.

Suggested Duration
12 months, then as needed

Nitric Oxide Activator
Use daily to support healthy cognitive function.

Frankincense
Apply 3-6 drops to bottoms of feet morning and evening to encourage heavy metal detox, and for cognitive support.

Nourishing Blend
Rub 2-4 drops along spine nightly.

Peppermint & Rosemary
Diffuse daily to stimulate mental activity.

Also Try
- Balancing Blend
- Lemon
- Moringa Super Powder

Back, Neck & Shoulder Pain

Reduces pain and inflammation; restores mobility.

Suggested Duration
4 weeks, then as needed

Optimal Aging Blend
Use daily to reduce inflammation and promote healthy muscular function.

Nitric Oxide Activator
Use daily to encourage circulation in problematic areas.

Soothing Blend
Massage a few drops into painful areas as needed.

Marjoram & Helichrysum
Massage 2 drops each into muscles to mend and restore damage.

Also Try
- Massage Blend
- Frankincense
- Black Pepper

Protocols

Bathroom Spray

Neutralizes bathroom odors without chemical fragrances.

Lemongrass, Lime, Grapefruit
Add 10 drops each to glass spray bottle (not plastic). Fill the remaining with water. Add a bit of rubbing alcohol/vodka to eliminate the need to shake before use.

Also Try
- Tea Tree
- Juniper Berry
- Purifying Blend
- Slimming Blend

Blood Pressure (high)

Helps lower high blood pressure; promotes proper circulation.

Suggested Duration
4-8 weeks, then as needed

Nitric Oxide Activator
Use daily to dilate blood vessels and promote circulation.

Cypress, Ylang Ylang, Marjoram
Rub a drop of each onto bottoms of feet each morning.

Frankincense, Ylang Ylang, Marjoram, Lemon
Take 1-2 drops of each in a capsule daily.

Also Try
- Premium Tea
- Roman Chamomile

Bronchitis/Pneumonia

Reduces coughing; boosts immune system; combats respiratory infection.

Suggested Duration
5-10 days

Extreme Moringa Energy
Use daily to boost immune system.

Lime, Rosemary, Scotch Pine
Rub 2 drops each onto chest, upper back, and bottoms of feet several times a day.

Balsam Fir & Lemon
Gargle a drop of each with water for 30 seconds, then swallow.

Also Try
- Thyme
- Oregano
- Respiratory Blend

Protocols

Cancer

Promotes healthy cellular apoptosis and cellular function.

Suggested Duration
6-12 months

Nourishing Blend
Rub 2-4 drops along spine and bottoms of feet twice daily.

Frankincense
Rub 3-5 drops as close to the affected area as possible 3x/daily.

Moringa Super Powder
Use daily to restore nutrients to healthy cells.

Also Try
- Alkaline water & diet
- Helichrysum
- Sandalwood
- Geranium

Candida

Combats fungus overgrowth in gut; allows for healthy bacterial growth.

Suggested Duration
4 weeks

Premium Tea
Use tea twice daily to flush toxins from gut and organs.

Immunity-Boosting Blend
Take 3-6 drops in a capsule 3x/daily to eliminate candida in gut.

Lemon
Drink a couple drops in water 3x/day.

Also Try
- Detoxification Blend
- Oregano
- Thyme
- Tea Tree

Canker Sores

Combats viral and bacterial infection; reduces pain.

Suggested Duration
As needed

Extreme Moringa Capsules
Use to boost immune system.

Frankincense & Tea Tree
Apply a drop of each diluted to the outside of cheek, over canker sore.

Black Pepper & Tea Tree
Use a drop of each diluted directly on canker sore.

Also Try
- Protecting Blend
- Clove
- Lime

Carpet Deodorizer

Eliminates carpet odors from food and pets naturally.

Suggested Duration
As needed

Purifying Blend, Lemon, Lime, Tea Tree
Combine 5 drops each with 1 cup baking soda. Rub evenly throughout carpet, and let sit for 12-24 hours before vacuuming.

Also Try
- Grapefruit
- Bergamot
- Scotch Pine

Celiac's Disease

Promotes nutrient absorption; calms digestive system.

Suggested Duration
Ongoing

PM Craving Control Caps
Use regularly to promote healthy digestion.

Premium Tea
Use a few times weekly to detox gut.

Digestive Support Blend
Take 2-4 drops internally, or rub on outside of stomach at the onset of pain.

Helichrysum
Take 2-4 drops internally daily to help heal the gut.

Also Try
- Cinnamon
- Frankincense
- Copaiba

Cholesterol (high)

Helps return high cholesterol levels back to normal levels.

Suggested Duration
4-6 weeks

Nitric Oxide Activator
Use daily to promote healthy circulation.

Marjoram & Lemongrass
Take 2 drops each in a capsule daily.

Cypress & Balancing Blend
Rub 2 drops each into bottoms of feet each morning.

Also Try
- Daily Tea
- Slimming Blend
- Lemon
- Clary Sage
- Helichrysum

Cold Sores

Combats viral infection; promotes skin healing and pain relief.

Suggested Duration
As needed

Extreme Moringa Energy
Use daily to enhance immune system.

Tea Tree & Black Pepper
Apply a drop of each diluted several times during symptoms.

Frankincense or Helichrysum
Apply a drop diluted between Melissa & Black Pepper to promote skin healing.

Also Try
- Atlas Cedarwood
- Protecting Blend

Colds

Provides antiviral respiratory support.

Suggested Duration
5-10 days

Extreme Moringa Energy
Use daily to enhance immune system.

Protecting Blend
Take 2-4 drops in water or capsule 3x/day.

Protecting Blend, Black Pepper, Tea Tree
Rub 1-2 drops on bottoms of feet 3x/day.

Respiratory Blend
Rub onto chest or diffuse as needed.

Also Try
- Rosemary
- Lime
- Extreme Moringa Capsules

Cough

Calms coughing; promotes restful breathing.

Suggested Duration
As needed

Nitric Oxide Activator
Use daily to promote cardiovascular health.

Extreme Moringa Energy
Use to enhance immune system.

Peppermint, Rosemary, & Lime
Rub 2 drops of each onto chest and bottoms of feet.

Respiratory Blend
Diffuse several drops.

Also Try
- Eucalyptus
- Respiration Blend
- Scotch Pine

Crohn's

Reduces inflammation and swelling in the bowels.

Suggested Duration
6 months

Premium Tea
Use regularly to provide calming to the gut.

Digestive Support Blend
Take 1-3 drops in water or a capsule as needed.

Helichrysum
Drink 1-2 drops in water or a capsule daily to promote healing in the gut.

Also Try
- Daily Digestive Blend
- Ginger
- Marjoram

Deodorant (body)

Helps manage bacteria and odor-causing toxicity.

Suggested Duration
4 weeks, then as needed

Premium Tea
Use regularly to flush toxicity from the body.

Detoxification Blend
Use 1-3 drops internally, or rub onto the bottoms of feet each morning.

Purifying Blend
Use diluted with carrier oil under arms after showering.

Also Try
- Tea Tree
- Atlas Cedarwood
- Weight Control Blend

Depression

Improves brain chemistry; supports healthy hormone production.

Suggested Duration
3-6 months, then as needed

Moringa Super Powder
Use daily to provide nutrients to the brain and hormone-producing systems.

Orange & Peppermint
Inhale a drop of each from cupped hands for a mood boost throughout the day.

Frankincense
Press a drop to the roof of the mouth 2-3 times daily.

Also Try
- Lime
- Vitality-Boosting Blend
- Extreme Moringa Capsules
- Optimal Aging Formula

Protocols

Detox

Helps eliminate toxicity and free up filtering organs.

Suggested Duration
4 weeks

Premium Tea
Use daily to gently facilitate detox process.

Detoxification Blend
Take 1-3 drops in water or a capsule daily.

Lemon
Drink 1-3 drops in water throughout the day.

Coriander & Juniper Berry
Rub 2-4 drops on bottoms of feet and over liver & kidneys once daily.

Also Try
- Frankincense
- Geranium

Diabetes (type 1)

Stimulates cellular maintenance; helps balance blood sugar.

Suggested Duration
3-6 months, then as needed

Optimal Aging Formula
Use daily as directed.

Nitric Oxide Activator
Use daily as directed.

Rosemary, Coriander, Cinnamon
Take 1 drop each in a capsule daily. Also rub diluted over pancreas.

Also Try
- Nourishing Blend
- Moringa Super Powder
- Juniper Berry
- Bergamot

Diabetes (type 2)

Helps balance blood sugar; supports pancreas.

Suggested Duration
3-6 months, then as needed

Moringa Super Powder
Use daily to provide nutrients to pancreas.

Coriander, Cinnamon, Juniper Berry
Take 1-2 drops each in a capsule daily.

Detoxification Blend
Rub 2 drops over pancreas daily.

Also Try
- Slimming Blend
- Weight Control Blend
- Daily Tea

Digestive Issues

Relieves inflammation, gas, and discomfort in the digestive system.

Suggested Duration
2-4 weeks, then as needed

Daily Tea
Use tea to promote calm in the gut.

Daily Digestive Blend
Take 2 softgels twice daily.

Frankincense & Peppermint
Use 2 drops in water or a capsule to ease pain the gut. Also rub on outside of stomach.

Also Try
- Ginger
- Fennel
- Digestive Support Blend
- Moringa Super Powder

Eczema/Dermatitis

Relieves itchiness; promotes skin repair

Suggested Duration
2-4 weeks

Optimal Aging Formula
Use daily to provide nutrients to skin.

Skin-Enriching Blend
Apply 2-4 drops diluted to affected areas once daily.

Detoxification Blend
Rub 2-4 drops to bottoms of feet morning and night.

Also Try
- Tea Tree
- Frankincense
- Helichrysum
- Lavender

Fatigue

Supports adrenals, micro-circulation, and alertness.

Suggested Duration
4 weeks, then as needed

Nitric Oxide Activator
Use daily to increase circulation and nutrient distribution.

Extreme Moringa Energy
Use to daily to naturally stimulate the body and mind.

Peppermint & Rosemary
Apply 2 drops to the bottoms of feet daily. Inhale from cupped hands as needed.

Lemon & Grapefruit
Drink 2-4 drops in water throughout the day.

Also Try
- Vitality-Boosting Blend
- Extreme Moringa Caps
- Limitless Energy Powder

Protocols

Fibromyalgia

Decreases inflammation; promotes healthy cellular function.

Suggested Duration
2-6 months, then as needed

Optimal Aging Blend
Use daily to help manage inflammation.

Nourishing Blend
Apply 2-4 drops along spine or bottoms of feet nightly.

Daily Cell Health Blend
Take 2 softgels twice daily for cellular support.

Soothing Blend
Massage into inflamed areas as often as needed.

Also Try
- Frankincense
- Detoxification Blend
- Orange
- Moringa Super Powder

Flu Bomb

Combats viruses; boosts immune system; supports respiratory system.

Suggested Duration
5-10 days.

Extreme Moringa Energy
Use daily to boost immune system.

Nitric Oxide Activator
Use daily to deliver oxygen and nutrients throughout body.

Oregano, Tea Tree, Protecting Blend, Lemon
Take 1-2 drops each in a capsule 3x/day.

Respiratory Blend
Inhale 1-2 drops from cupped hands, or diffuse several drops.

Also Try
- Black Pepper
- Thyme

Heartburn

Balances stomach acid; eases pain of indigestion.

Suggested Duration
As needed

Moringa Super Powder
Use daily to support healthy digestion.

Daily Tea
Use to de-stress stomach.

Digestive Support Blend
Drink 1-2 drops in water or a capsule.

Peppermint
Rub a drop onto outside of stomach at the onset of heartburn.

Also Try
- Daily Digestive Blend
- Ginger
- Fennel

Protocols

Immune Boost

Provides antibacterial and antiviral support; boosts immune system.

Suggested Duration
4 weeks

Extreme Moringa Energy
Use daily to enhance immune system.

Protecting Blend, Black Pepper, Tea Tree
Rub a drop of each onto bottoms of feet daily.

Daily Cell Health Blend
Take 1 softgel twice daily.

Also Try
- Frankincense
- Thyme
- Extreme Moringa Capsules
- Optimal Aging Formula

Infertility

Supports the reproductive system and proper hormone production.

Suggested Duration
2-6 months

Optimal Aging Formula
Use daily to balance and maintain body systems.

Nitric Oxide Activator
Use to deliver oxygen and nutrients to reproductive organs.

Moringa Super Powder
Use daily to provide needed nutrients.

Men's/Women's Daily Balancing Blend
Use twice daily.

Clary Sage
Rub 2 drops over bladder and onto bottoms of feet daily.

Irritable Bowels

Calms chronic digestive irritation and diarrhea.

Suggested Duration
2-4 weeks

Moringa Super Powder
Use daily to promote healthy digestion,.

Daily Tea
Use to calm the gut.

Daily Digestive Blend
Take 2 softgels twice daily.

Stress Control Blend
Inhale 2 drops from cupped hands several times daily.

Also Try
- Digestive Support Blend
- Fennel
- Peppermint

Protocols

Libido (low sex drive)

Inspires inhibited sex drive.

Suggested Duration
2 weeks, then as needed

Nitric Oxide Activator
Use daily, especially before intimacy.

Ylang Ylang
Rub a drop onto pulse points daily.

Cinnamon
Use 1-2 drops in water throughout the day.

Men's/Women's Daily Balancing Blend
Take 1 softgel twice daily.

Also Try
- Clary Sage
- Extreme Moringa Energy

Lupus

Reduces inflammation; supports cellular function and healthy DNA.

Suggested Duration
6-12 months

Optimal Aging Formula
Use daily to help manage inflammation.

Moringa Super Powder
Use daily to provide needed nutrients.

Nourishing Blend
Rub 2-4 drops onto spine nightly.

Daily Cell Health Blend
Take 1 softgel twice daily.

Soothing Blend & Frankincense
Massage into inflamed areas as needed.

Also Try
- Restorative Blend

Lyme Disease

Provides strong antibacterial support; reduces inflammation.

Suggested Duration
2 week intervals with 1 week rest in-between as needed

Moringa Super Powder
Use daily to support immune system.

Optimal Aging Formula
Use daily to reduce inflammation.

Cinnamon, Oregano, Thyme, Clove
Take 2 drops each in a capsule twice daily.

Frankincense & Black Pepper
Massage 1-2 drops over lymph nodes daily.

Also Try
- Protecting Blend
- Extreme Moringa Capsules

Menopause

Aids in hormone and mood balance; calms hot flashes.

Suggested Duration
4 months, then as needed

Women's Daily Balancing Blend
Take 1 softgel twice daily.

Moringa Super Powder
Use daily to provide nutrients for healthy hormone production.

Peppermint
Apply a drop to back of neck to ease hot flashes.

Also Try
- Clary Sage
- Ylang Ylang
- Geranium

Menstruation

Balances mood and hormones during menstruation.

Suggested Duration
2 weeks as needed

Women's Daily Balancing Blend
Take 1 softgel twice daily.

Monthly Blend
Rub 1-3 drops over lower abdomen and on wrists.

Balancing Blend
Apply a drop behind ears to stabilize mood as needed.

Also Try
- Moringa Super Powder
- Clary Sage
- Comforting Blend

Mononucleosis

Provides antiviral support; restores energy levels.

Suggested Duration
2-4 weeks.

Extreme Moringa Energy
Use to boost immune system and restore energy.

Thyme, Oregano, Protecting Blend
Take 1-2 drops each in a capsule 3x/day.

Frankincense & Black Pepper
Rub 2 drops each onto bottoms of feet in the mornings.

Also Try
- Extreme Moringa Capsules
- Cinnamon
- Immunity-Boosting Blend

Protocols

Muscle Aches

Reduces inflammation, spasms, and pain in muscles.

Suggested Duration
2 weeks, then as needed.

Optimal Aging Blend
Use daily to help ease inflammation.

Nitric Oxide Activator
Use daily to increase circulation and deliver oxygen to muscles.

Massage Blend
Massage 2-4 drops into aching muscles 3x/day.

Frankincense & Lemon
Take 1-2 drops each in water or a capsule 2x/day.

Also Try
- Moringa Super Powder
- Soothing Blend
- Cypress
- Restorative Blend

Pregnancy (postnatal)

Promotes pain relief, tissue healing, and emotional support after birth.

Suggested Duration
4-8 weeks

Moringa Super Powder
Use daily to provide nutrients for healthy hormones and recovery.

Helichrysum, Frankincense, Lavender
Apply 2 drops each diluted to areas with tearing 3x/day.

Ylang Ylang
Diffuse for mood balancing.

Basil or Fennel
Massage diluted around breasts to stimulate milk.

Helichrysum, Myrrh, Lavender
Massage 2 drops each diluted into stretch mark areas.

Pregnancy (prenatal)

Relieves pregnancy sickness; provides vital nutrients and emotional support.

Suggested Duration
9 months

Moringa Super Powder
Use daily to provide crucial nutrients.

Digestive Support Blend
Drink 2 drops in water or a capsule, or rub 2 drops over stomach to ease nausea.

Comforting Blend
Inhale 1-2 drops from cupped hands, or diffuse to elevate mood.

Also Try
- Women's Daily Balancing Blend
- Ginger
- Stress Control Blend

Psoriasis

Relieves itchy, swollen skin; promotes proper immune system function.

Suggested Duration
4-8 weeks

Optimal Aging Formula
Use to reduce inflammation.

Helichrysum, Frankincense, Tea Tree, Lavender
Combine 10 drops each with carrier oil in a roller bottle. Apply 3x/day.

Nourishing Blend
Take 2-4 drops in water or a capsule twice daily.

Detoxification Blend
Rub 2-4 drops onto bottoms of feet each morning.

Also Try
- Skin-Enriching Blend
- Copaiba
- Atlas Cedarwood

Shingles

Provides antiviral support, along with viral detox.

Suggested Duration
4 weeks, then as needed

Extreme Moringa Energy
Use daily to enhance immune system.

Tea Tree, Frankincense, Black Pepper
Take 1-2 each in a capsule 3x/day.

Frankincense & Lavender
Apply 2 drops each diluted to affected areas.

Detoxification Blend
Rub 2-4 drops onto bottoms of feet each morning.

Also Try
- Lime
- Protecting Blend
- Atlas Cedarwood

Sinus Bomb

Helps combat sinus infection.

Suggested Duration
5-10 days

Extreme Moringa Energy
Use daily to enhance immune system.

Myrrh, Oregano, Frankincense, Lemon
Combine 10 drops each (3 drops of Oregano) with carrier oil in roller bottle. Apply carefully over cheek bones and brow, avoiding eyes 3-5x/day.

Immunity-Boosting Blend
Take 1-2 drops in a capsule 3x/day.

Also Try
- Respiratory Blend
- Oregano
- Thyme
- Extreme Moringa Capsules

Protocols

Sleep Apnea

Promotes open airways and more meaningful sleep.

Suggested Duration
Ongoing

Nitric Oxide Activator
Use daily to open blood vessels and increase oxygenation.

Respiration Blend
Diffuse 5-10 drops next to bedside at night. Also apply to sinus reflex points.

Protecting Blend
Gargle 2 drops with water for 30 seconds each night, then swallow.

Comforting Blend
Apply 2 drops to temples before bed.

Also Try
- Peppermint
- Rosemary

Sleep & Insomnia

Supports falling and staying asleep, and to wake feeling rested.

Suggested Duration
4 weeks, then as needed

Moringa Super Powder
Use daily to provide needed minerals for healthy neurological function.

Nitric Oxide Activator
Use daily as directed.

Lavender & Vetiver
Apply 1-2 drops to temples and bottoms of feet before bed. Diffuse several drops next to bedside.

Also Try
- Comforting Blend
- Atlas Cedarwood
- Roman Chamomile

Smoking Addiction

Helps curb cravings and smoking addiction; aids in detox.

Suggested Duration
6-12 weeks

PM Craving Control Caps
Use regularly to help reduce cravings.

Grapefruit
Drink 1-3 drops in water throughout the day.

Protecting Blend
Swish 2 drops with water immediately after eating.

Black Pepper
Apply 1 drop to big toes 2x/day. Also inhale or diffuse throughout the day.

Also Try
- Detoxification Blend
- Clove
- Premium Tea

Snoring

Promotes open airways during sleep.

Suggested Duration
Ongoing

Nitric Oxide Activator
Use daily to encourage good oxygenation.

Respiratory Blend
Diffuse 5-10 drops near bedside at night. Also apply t chest, throat, and lung reflex points.

Protecting Blend
Gargle 2 drops with water for 30 seconds before bed, then swallow.

Lemon
Drink 1-3 drops in warm water before bed.

Also Try
- Scotch Pine
- Respiration Blend

Sore Throat

Relieves pain and soreness in throat; combats bacteria and viruses.

Suggested Duration
5-10 days

Extreme Moringa Energy
Use daily to enhance immune system.

Lemon (10 drops), Protecting blend (8), Helichrysum (2)
Combine in small glass spray bottle with carrier oil. Spray into back of throat as needed.

Lavender & Atlas Cedarwood
Massage 1-2 drops to outside of throat.

Also Try
- Black Pepper
- Thyme
- Extreme Moringa Capsules

Stress-Away

Reduces excess cortisol levels; balances emotions.

Suggested Duration
4 weeks, then as needed

Daily Tea
Use to calm cellular stress.

Stress Control Blend
Inhale 1-2 drops from cupped hands, or apply to pulse points as needed.

Frankincense & Lavender
Diffuse several drops throughout the day.

Also Try
- Comforting Blend
- Moringa Super Powder

Sunburn

Relieves discomfort from sunburn; promotes quicker healing.

Suggested Duration
3-7 days

Lavender & Helichrysum
Apply 2-4 drops with carrier oil or aloe to sunburnt skin 3-5x/day.

Peppermint
Add 5 drops to small glass spray bottle with water. Spritz onto school skin.

Also Try
- Moringa-enhanced skincare
- Atlas Cedarwood
- Copaiba
- Roman Chamomile

Thrush

Provides anti-fungal support; eases oral discomfort.

Suggested Duration
1-3 weeks

Lemon & Tea Tree
Combine 2 drops each with 1 Tbs of carrier oil. Apply with clean finger to child's gums and tongue 2-3x/day.

Lavender & Tea Tree
Massage diluted into bottoms of child's feet and on stomach daily.

Also Try
- Protecting Blend
- Geranium
- Extreme Moringa Energy

Thyroid (Hyper/Grave's)

Calms an overactive thyroid; balances thyroid hormones.

Suggested Duration
4-6 months

Premium Tea
Use to calm cellular stress.

Myrrh, Frankincense, Rosemary
Combine 10 drops each in roller bottle, and fill remaining with carrier oil. Apply over thyroid 3x/day.

Daily Cell Health Blend
Take 2 softgels 2x/day.

Also Try
- Lemongrass

Protocols

Thyroid
(Hypo/Hashimoto's)

Stimulates thyroid in order to produce proper hormones.

Suggested Duration
4-6 months

Extreme Moringa Capsules
Use to stimulate body and provide needed nutrients.

Clove, Myrrh, Lemongrass, Peppermint
Combine 10 drops each in roller bottle, fill remaining with carrier oil. Apply over thyroid 3-5x/day. Also take a drop of each in capsule 3x/day for first week.

Daily Cell Health Blend
Take 2 softgels 2x/day.

Also Try
- Bergamot
- Spearmint
- Nitric Oxide Activator

Weight-loss

Stimulates metabolism; curbs appetite; aids in detox.

Suggested Duration
4-12 weeks

AM Exercise Enhancing Caps
Use daily to enhance and inspire exercise.

Extreme Moringa Energy
Use daily to supply needed fuel and nutrients.

Advanced Thermogenic Caps
Use to increase basal metabolic rate.

Weight Control Blend
Drink 2-4 drops in water throughout the day.

Also Try
- Slimming Blend
- Grapefruit
- PM Craving Control Caps

Workout Support

Provides pre- and post workout support; supports building muscle.

Suggested Duration
Ongoing

Extreme Moringa Energy
Use daily to supply needed fuel and nutrients.

Plant Protein
Use after workouts and meals to help build lean muscle.

Pre-, During, and Post-Workout Powders
Use to maximize the efficacy of workout routines.

Also Try
- Vitality-Boosting Blend
- Respiratory Blend
- Limitless Energy Powder
- Soothing Blend

Bibliography

Aromatic Science. AromaticScience, LLC. Web. July, 2017. <www.aromaticscience.com>

Enlighten Alternative Healing. Emotions and Essential Oils: A Modern Resource for Healing: Emotional Reference Guide. 3rd ed., Enlighten Alternative Healing, 2016.

Harding, Jennie: The Essential Oils Handbook. Duncan Baird Publishers Ltd, 2008.

Lawless, Julia: The Encyclopedia of Essential Oils: The Complete Guide to the Use of Aromatic Oils In Aromatherapy, Herbalism, Health, and Well Being. Conari Press, 2013.

Louis, Joy: Moringa The Miracle Tree: Nature's Most Powerful Superfood Revealed. Joy Louis Books, 2014.

Mind Body Green. MindBodyGreen, LLC. Web. December 2015. <mindbodygreen.com>

Schiller, Carol & Schiller, David: The Aromatherapy Encyclopedia: A Concise Guide to Over 395 Plant Oils. Basic Health Publications Inc, 2008.

Schnaubelt, Kurt. The Healing Intelligence of Essential Oils: the Science of Advanced Aromatherapy. Healing Arts Press, 2011.

Tisserand, Robert, et al. Essential Oil Safety: A Guide for Health Care Professionals. 2nd ed., Churchill Livingstone/Elsevier, 2014.

Worwood, Valerie Ann. The Complete Book of Essential Oils and Aromatherapy, Revised and Expanded: Over 800 Natural, Nontoxic, and Fragrant Recipes to Create Health, Beauty, And Safe Home and Work Environments. New World Library, 2016.

Shareable Protocols

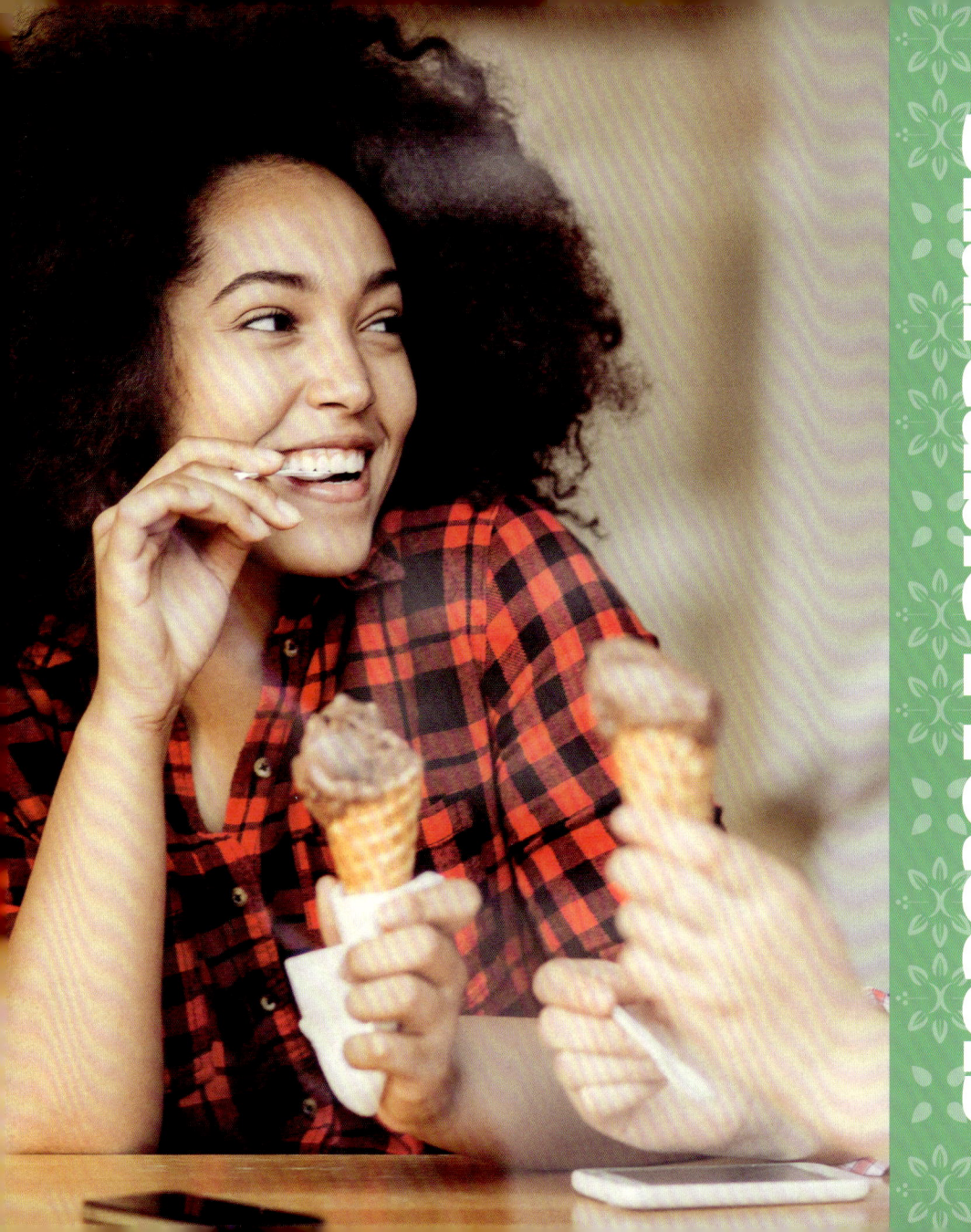

ADD/ADHD

Increases focus and concentration, supports healthy brain chemistry.

Suggested Duration
Ongoing

Nitric Oxide Activator
Use daily as directed for oxygenation.

Moringa Super Powder
Use daily to supply nutrients to brain.

Vetiver
Apply a dab behind ears as needed.

Restorative Blend
Inhale 1-2 drops from cupped hands.

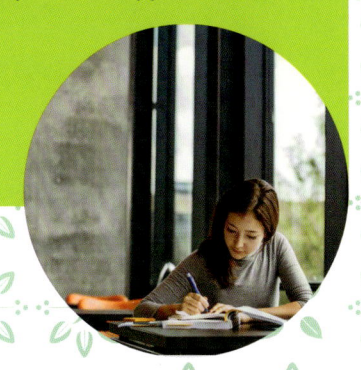

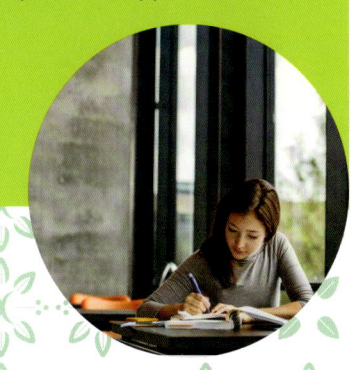

"Health is the greatest gift, contentment is the greatest wealth, faithfulness the best relationship."

-Buddha

Find more protocols like this in the book
GURULIFE

"A calm mind brings inner strength and self-confidence."

-Dalai Lama

Find more protocols like this in the book
GURULIFE

Allergies

Reduces histamine response and boosts immune system.

Suggested Duration
4-8 weeks to begin, then as needed

Extreme Moringa Energy
Use daily to boost immune response.

Lemon, Lavender, Peppermint
Put 1 drop each under the tongue during flare-ups. Drink water after 30 seconds.

Respiratory Blend
Inhale 1-3 drops from cupped hands, and rub carefully over bridge of nose.

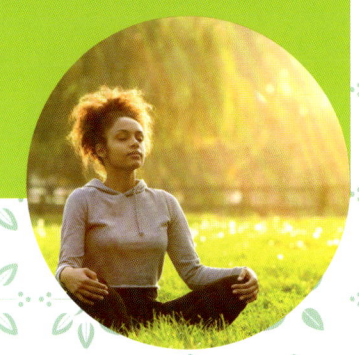

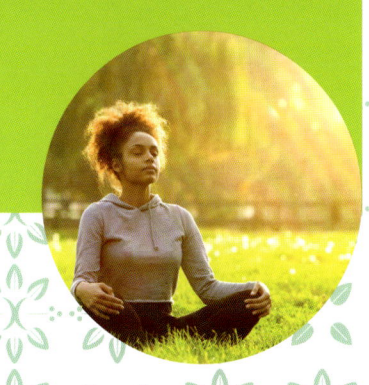

"In three words I can sum up everything I've learned about life: It goes on."

-Robert Frost

Find more protocols like this in the book
GURULIFE

"As for butter versus margarine, I trust cows more than chemists."

-Joan Gussow

Find more protocols like this in the book
GURULIFE

Anxiety & Stress

Reduces stress levels; promotes a sense of calm, security, and focus.

Suggested Duration
3-6 months, then as needed

Premium Tea
Use nightly to ease stress from the day.

Stress Control Blend
Carry with you, and inhale from cupped hands often as needed for mood support.

Balancing Blend
Apply 2 drops to the bottoms of feet each morning to start the day grounded.

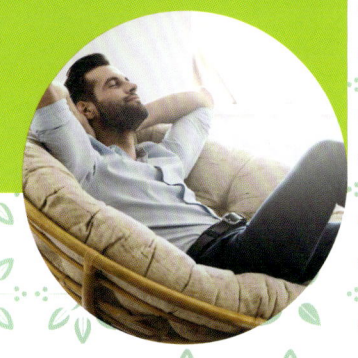

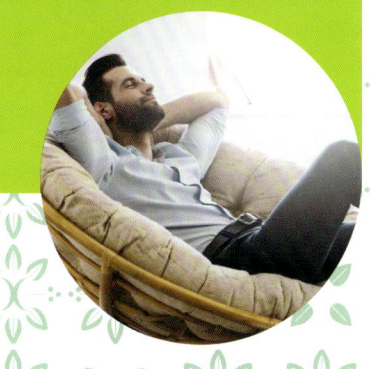

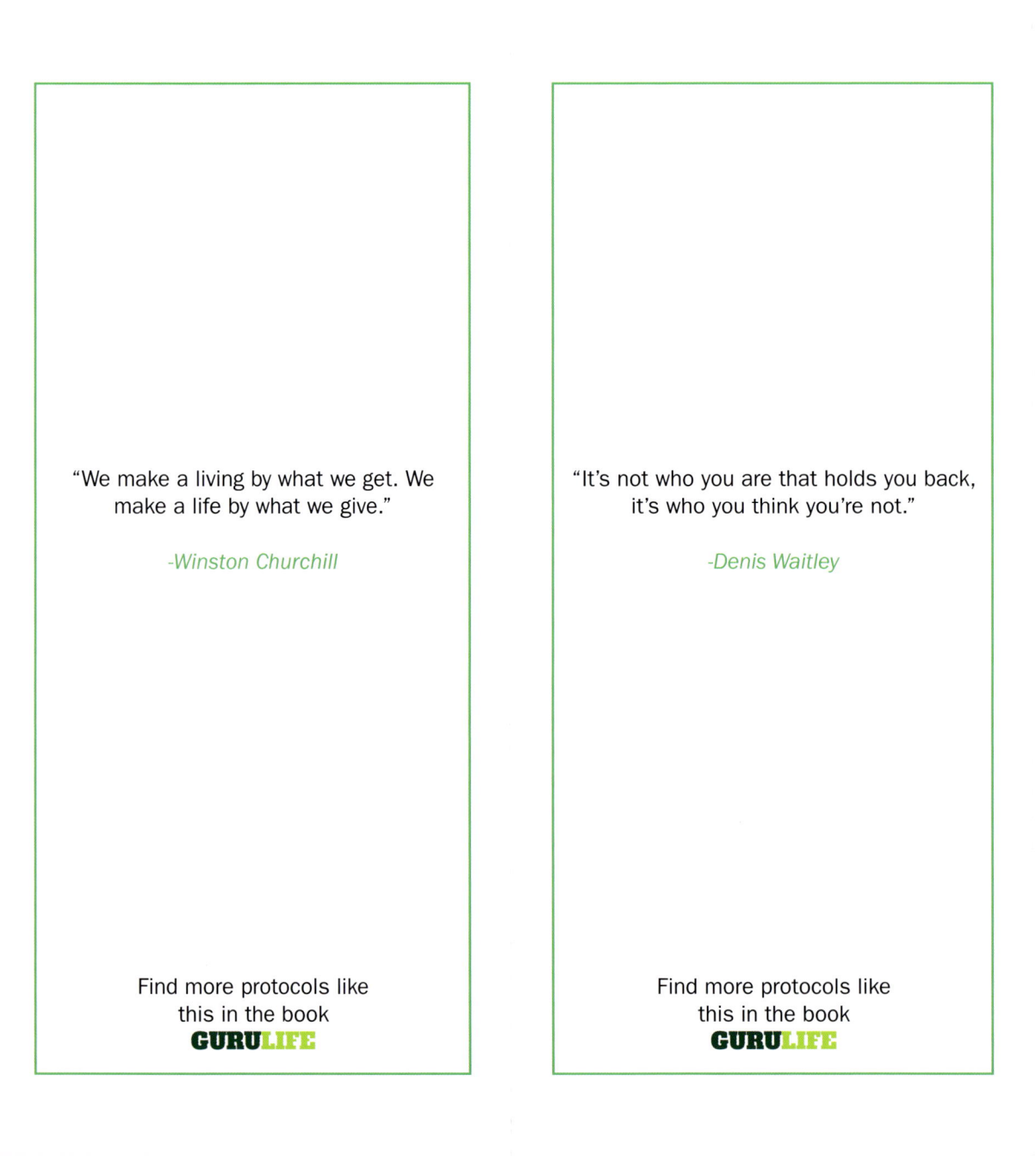

"We make a living by what we get. We make a life by what we give."

-Winston Churchill

Find more protocols like
this in the book
GURULIFE

"It's not who you are that holds you back, it's who you think you're not."

-Denis Waitley

Find more protocols like
this in the book
GURULIFE

Back, Neck, & Shoulders

Reduces pain and inflammation; restores mobility.

Suggested Duration
4 weeks, then as needed

Optimal Aging Blend
Use daily to reduce inflammation.

Nitric Oxide Activator
Use daily to encourage circulation and oxygenation to problematic areas.

Soothing Blend
Massage a few drops into painful areas as needed.

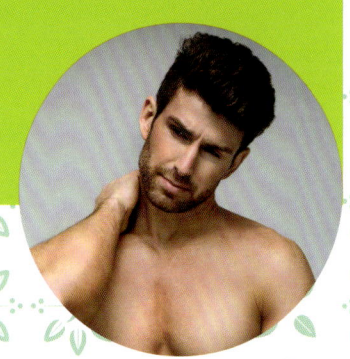

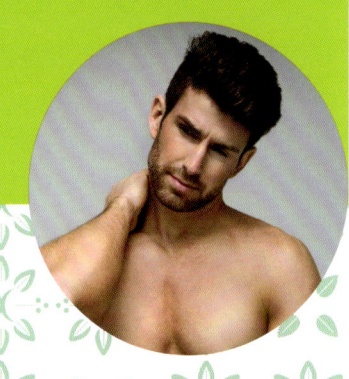

"Nothing is impossible. The word itself says *I'm possible*."

-*Audrey Hepburn*

Find more protocols like this in the book
GURULIFE

"If you obey all the rules, you miss all the fun."

-*Katharine Hepburn*

Find more protocols like this in the book
GURULIFE

Colds

Provides antiviral respiratory support.

Suggested Duration
5-10 days

Extreme Moringa Energy
Use daily to enhance immune system.

Protecting Blend
Take 2-4 drops in water or a capsule three times daily.

Respiratory Blend
Rub a few drops onto chest, inhale from cupped hand, or diffuse as needed.

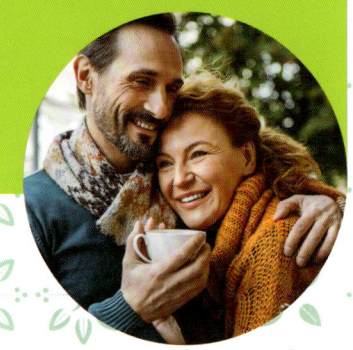

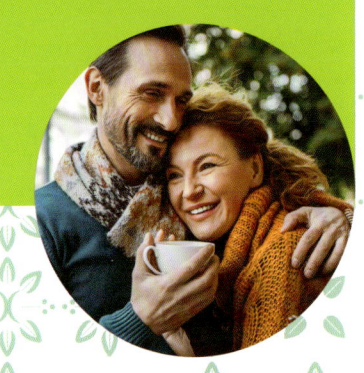

"Motivation will always beat mere talent."

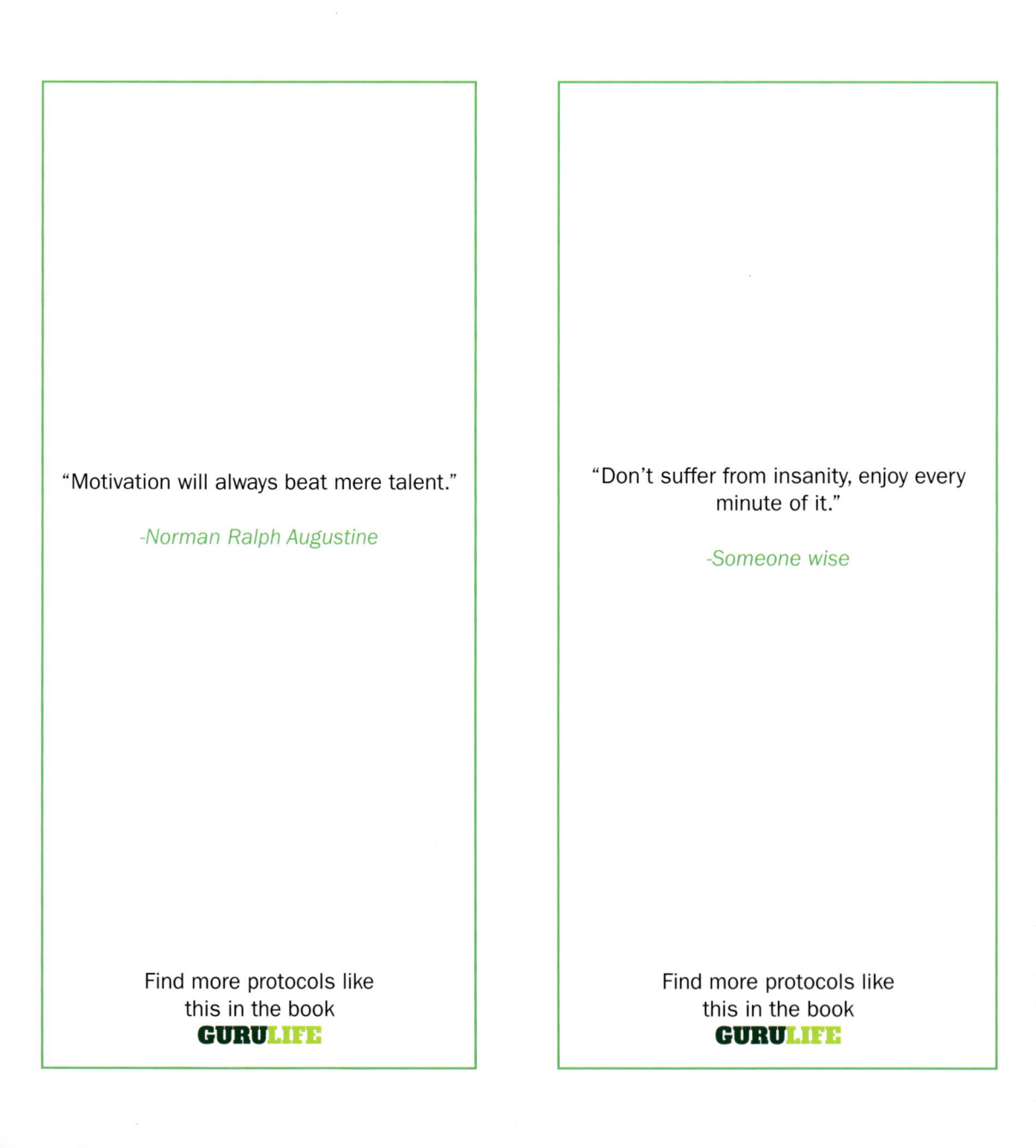

-Norman Ralph Augustine

Find more protocols like
this in the book
GURULIFE

"Don't suffer from insanity, enjoy every minute of it."

-Someone wise

Find more protocols like
this in the book
GURULIFE

Depression

Improves brain chemistry, supports healthy hormone production.

Suggested Duration
3-6 months, then as needed

Moringa Super Powder
Use Moringa daily as directed to provide needed nutrients.

Stress-Control Blend
Carry with you, and inhale from cupped hands often as needed for mood support.

Frankincense
Put a drop under the tongue 1-3x/day.

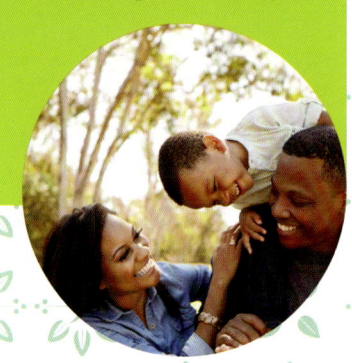

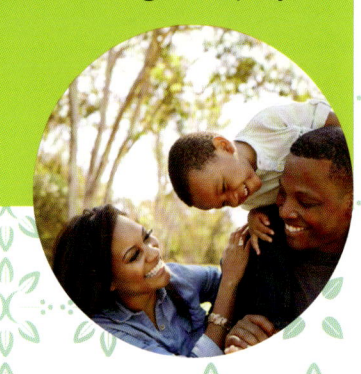

"Your imagination is your preview to life's coming attractions."

-Albert Einstein

Find more protocols like this in the book
GURULIFE

"Success is getting what you want. Happiness is wanting everything you get."

-Dale Carnegie

Find more protocols like this in the book
GURULIFE

Digestive Issues

Relieves inflammation, gas, and discomfort in the digestive system.

Suggested Duration
2-4 weeks, then as needed

Moringa Super Powder
Use Moringa to support healthy digestion.

Daily Digestive Blend
Take 2 softgels twice daily.

Frankincense & Peppermint
Drink 2 drops in water, or rub on outside of stomach to ease stomach pain.

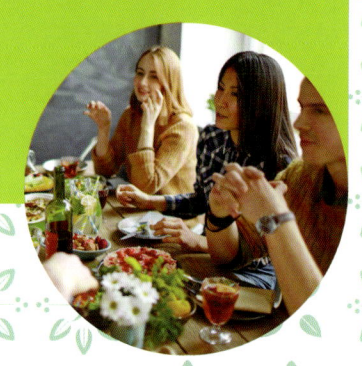

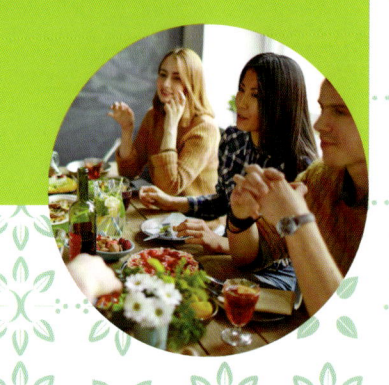

"People often say that motivation doesn't last. Well, neither does bathing; that's why we recommend it daily."

-Zig Ziglar

Find more protocols like this in the book
GURULIFE

"A fit, healthy body - that is the best fashion statement."

-Jess C. Scott

Find more protocols like this in the book
GURULIFE

Fatigue

Supports adrenals, micro-circulation, and alertness.

Suggested Duration
4 weeks, then as needed

Extreme Moringa Energy
Use daily to provide natural fuel.

Nitric Oxide Activator
Use daily for circulation & oxygenation.

Peppermint & Rosemary
Apply 2 drops to the bottoms of feet daily. Inhale from cupped hands as needed.

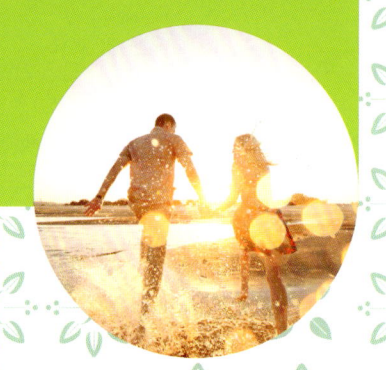

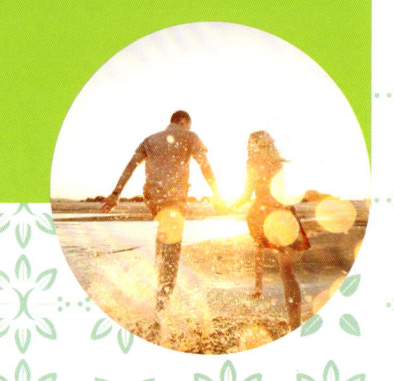

"You live only once, but if you do it right, once is enough."

-Mae West

Find more protocols like this in the book
GURULIFE

"A healthy attitude is contagious, but don't wait to catch it from others; be a carrier."

-Tom Stoppard

Find more protocols like this in the book
GURULIFE

Flu Bomb

Combats viruses; boosts immune system; supports respiratory system.

Suggested Duration
5-10 Days

Extreme Moringa Energy
Use daily to enhance immune system.

Immunity-Boosting Blend
Take 2-4 drops in a capsule 3x/day.

Respiratory Blend
Inhale 1-2 drops from cupped hands, or diffuse several drops.

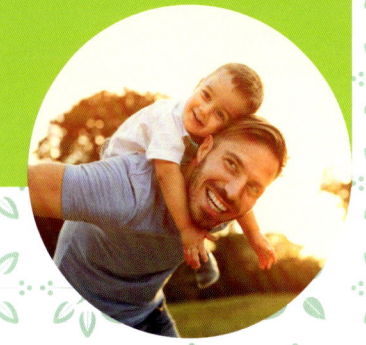

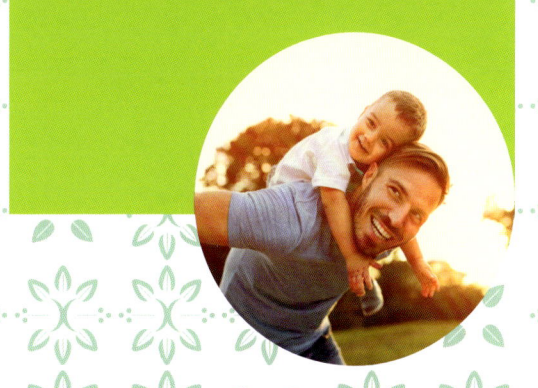

"If you're happy, if you're feeling good, then nothing else matters."

-Robin Wright

Find more protocols like
this in the book
GURULIFE

"The produce manager is more important to my children's health than the pediatrician."

-Meryl Streep

Find more protocols like
this in the book
GURULIFE

Sleep & Insomnia

Supports falling and staying asleep, and to wake feeling rested.

Suggested Duration
4 weeks, then as needed

Moringa Super Powder
Use Moringa daily to provide nutrients to neurological system.

Nitric Oxide Activator
Use daily to promote oxygenation and neurological function.

Lavender & Vetiver
Apply 1-2 drops to temples and bottoms of feet before bed.

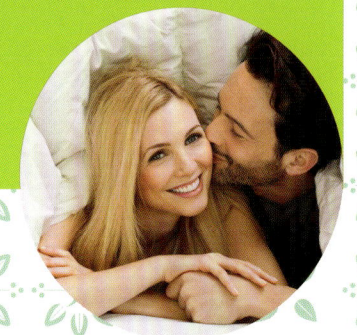

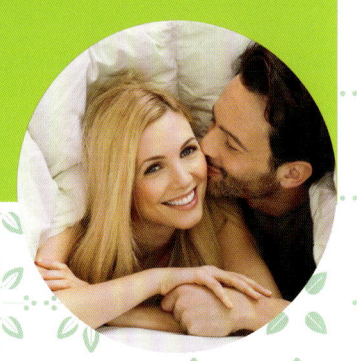

"Rest when you're weary. Refresh and renew yourself, your body, your mind, your spirit. Then get back to work."

-Ralph Marston

Find more protocols like this in the book
GURULIFE

"I believe that the greatest gift you can give your family and the world is a healthy you."

-Joyce Meyer

Find more protocols like this in the book
GURULIFE